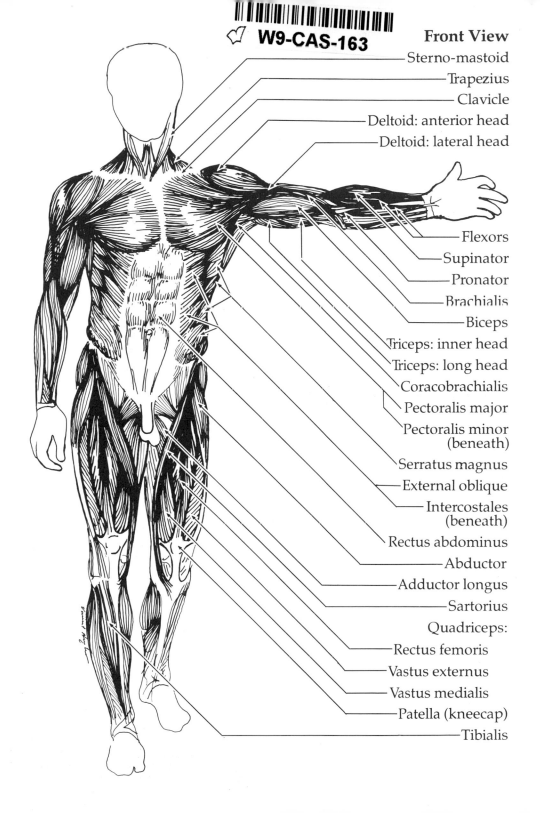

Front View

Sterno-mastoid

Trapezius

Clavicle

Deltoid: anterior head

Deltoid: lateral head

Flexors

Supinator

Pronator

Brachialis

Biceps

Triceps: inner head

Triceps: long head

Coracobrachialis

Pectoralis major

Pectoralis minor (beneath)

Serratus magnus

External oblique

Intercostales (beneath)

Rectus abdominus

Abductor

Adductor longus

Sartorius

Quadriceps:

Rectus femoris

Vastus externus

Vastus medialis

Patella (kneecap)

Tibialis

Rear View

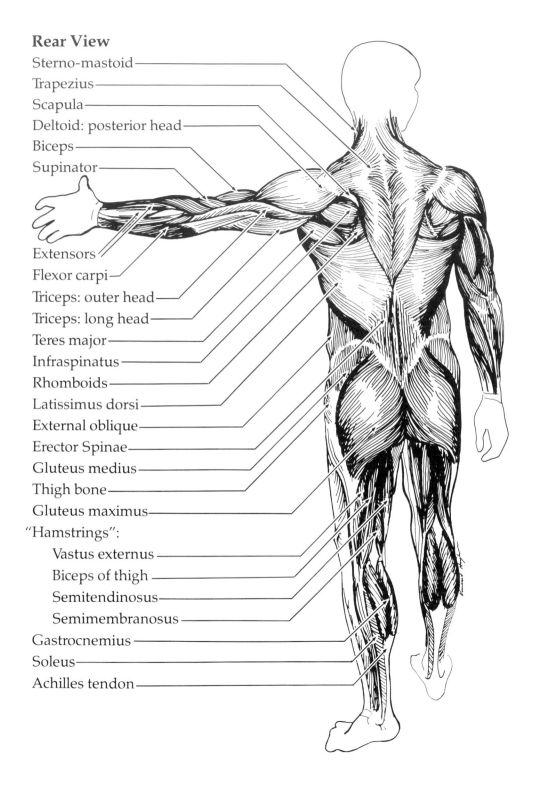

Sterno-mastoid
Trapezius
Scapula
Deltoid: posterior head
Biceps
Supinator

Extensors
Flexor carpi
Triceps: outer head
Triceps: long head
Teres major
Infraspinatus
Rhomboids
Latissimus dorsi
External oblique
Erector Spinae
Gluteus medius
Thigh bone
Gluteus maximus
"Hamstrings":
    Vastus externus
    Biceps of thigh
    Semitendinosus
    Semimembranosus
Gastrocnemius
Soleus
Achilles tendon

35 and HOLDING

COMPLETE CONDITIONING FOR THE ADULT MALE

Pete Broccoletti

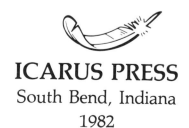

ICARUS PRESS

South Bend, Indiana

1982

35 and Holding
Copyright © 1982 by Pete Broccoletti

Manufactured in the United States of America

Icarus Press, Inc.
Post Office Box 1225
South Bend, Indiana 46624

1 2 3 4 5 6 86 85 84 83 82

Library of Congress Cataloging in Publication Data

Broccoletti, Pete, 1942–

    35 & holding.

    Includes index.
    1. Weight lifting.   2. Physical fitness for men.
I. Title.   II. Title: Thirty-five and holding.
GV546.3.B76   796.4'1   82-2927
ISBN 0-89651-778-0   AACR2
ISBN 0-89651-779-9 (wirebound)

CONTENTS

To the memory of my grandfathers,
Orlando Broccoletti and Peter Lusardi,
whose lives were examples of the spirit
that made this country great.
And to the memory of my father, Harold Broccoletti,
and godfather, Joseph Spisso,
who were great family men, noted sportsmen,
and beloved by all who knew them.

INTRODUCTION

After thirty five years of age, your metabolism slows down and your testerone level, which helps to build muscle in men, continues to drop every year. Because of the slowing down of your metabolism as you grow older, your body fat accumulates easier. Therefore, in order to stay in tone, you either have to change your diet (which you probably should do anyway) or burn up more calories. Burning up more calories is much harder at 35 than at 20 because you have less time due to job and perhaps family responsibilities. When you were in school, you were probably playing sports of some sort, throwing the frisbee around, running to class, chasing after dates and partying more, which uses up a lot of calories. Now you just don't have the time to do all the things you might like to, such as hiking, biking, swimming, playing tennis or golf. (Now you just don't have the time to do all the things you might like to, such as hiking, biking, swimming, playing tennis or golf.) You have to be much more selective in utilizing your time, both in terms of what you enjoy the most and what will best serve you in keeping in shape.

Just because you are over 35 doesn't mean you have to have a pot belly or a big fat rear end or even a sagging chest. Many great bodybuilders of today are over 35: Frank Zane a Mr. Olympia, Bill Pearl almost 50 and still in championship shape, Ed Corney 48 and still competing, and the indominatable John Grimek, editor of *Muscular Development*, a former titleholder who is approaching 70 and still is powerful with a fine physique men 50 years younger would like to have. My mentor, Father Lange, B.H.B. of Notre Dame University, was still a powerhouse when I trained under him while he was in his 70s. When I visited him a couple of years before his death in 1968, he was 80 years old. That didn't deter him from working out with 100-pound dumbbells on the bench press for sets of 12 to 13 reps. or from doing curls with 60-pound dumbbells for 12 to 15 reps.

Obviously we all can't be John Grimeks, Fr. Langes, or Bill Pearls. However, the vast majority of you don't want to be, but just want to be

1

toned up, to tighten up that stomach, firm up that chest, tighten up your posterior, and tone your legs.

When you look better, you feel better. When you look better, you build self-confidence, which is important not just for your social life but in dealing with clients, patients, customers, and your peers.

The models in this book are almost all over 35 and still looking good. And they will all be improving the way they look, not going downhill just because they have reached 35. You can shape up and look good too. It just takes determination, work, and the right diet. Besides the extensive weight training part of this book, the flexibility chapter, and the all-important diet and nutrition section, I have included an aerobics chapter. Weight training is great for shaping you up, but it generally doesn't have the circular respiratory conditioning that you need. This conditioning is important to keep your heart in shape. How many people have you heard of that have had heart attacks in their 40s? This is also called cardiovascular conditioning which to an extent can be obtained by circuit weight training but not to the ideal extent that you are able to obtain from swimming or bicycling. In this book, for the first time, you have a complete physical-fitness manual (weight training, aerobics, diet) that will help to improve your health as well as make you look good.

As a word of caution I recommend that you get a complete physical from your doctor as well as a stress test before you start exercising. You should specifically ask him whether there are any limits on your weight training or aerobic activity. Be sure to bring up any old injuries you might have had and check them out. Then I recommend one month of progressive calisthentics, sit-ups, leg raises, push-ups, and chin-ups if you haven't been training in the last year. An ounce of prevention is worth a pound of cure, and it's better to go slowly in getting into your new regime than chance injuring yourself by going hog wild at first.

NUTRITION

Adelle Davis's greatest contribution to the American public may have been her statement that "you are what you eat." Although there are a few psychologists around that are now saying that what you eat reflects your personality, I am referring to the fact that the physical composition and condition of your body is determined by what you eat. Good health starts in your kitchen. If you eat an unbalanced diet, you are going to develop vitamin or mineral deficiencies that could result in illness or at least a poor skin condition, fatigue, and irritability. If you eat a large amount of junk food, such as cake, cookies, candy, soda, potato chips, etc., you will not only most likely be overweight (at least one-third of Americans are) but have high blood pressure, making you a prime candidate for heart disease. You will also probably be experiencing the lows, depression, and irritability after your sugar high.

Although health-food stores are "in," just buying your supplies there is not automatically going to put you in good health. Unfortunately in many cases the food you buy in a health-food store might not be any better than that which you can buy in a regular grocery store. You should be careful in selecting what goods you buy at such a store so that you are not throwing your money away or gaining a false sense of security from eating that food. In many cases you will be able to buy some products in a health-food store that are more healthy than in a supermarket. Some examples of this are specially prepared whole wheat bread, homemade yogurt, and fruit and vegetables organically grown rather than those dosed with possibly harmful chemicals. I always recommend eating fresh fruits and vegetables because they will provide more minerals and vitamins than those that are frozen or canned. I also recommend steaming your vegetables, since you retain more of the nutrients this way. Besides avoiding junk food, avoid white or American bread because the flour is too processed. Instead eat French, Italian, whole wheat (which is the most preferable), rye, or pumpernickel. Avoid all sugars if possible. They are empty calories that give you an artificial high and result in a crash. All isolated sugars do this. Allow your body to obtain the natural sugars or fructose from the fruits you eat rather than adding sugar to your diet. If you need a sweetener in your coffee or tea use an artificial sweetener (be sure to read the label though!). Instead of putting junk food into your system for a snack, eat some nutritional food like plain yogurt with a couple of teaspoons of wheat germ or sliced fruit mixed in. Try some anchovies or sardines (with the oil washed off) on wheat thins or cheese on wheat thins.

Now that you are starting to exercise and getting in shape again, nutrition is even more important to you. You need more nutrients to give you the energy to exercise, repair muscle tissues, and promote muscle growth. However, you could exercise two hours a day for six days a week and not notice significant results if you are not eating correctly. An adult man needs about 2,500 calories a day in well-balanced meals to function properly. I will talk more about calories when I deal with diets later in this chapter. The foods we need include proteins, fats, carbohydrates, mineral salts, vitamins, and water. Generally, your diet while you are in training should be high in *complex* carbohydrates (60%), obtained primarily from vegetables and fruits; high in protein (25%), obtained from eggs, fowl, low-fat dairy products, and occasionally from lean meats; and low in fats (15%), easily obtained from lean meats, eggs, low-fat dairy products, and vegetables in your normal diet. This is neither a weight-loss nor a weight-gain diet.

Protein

Protein is incredibly important to weight-training athletes. It is the body's primary building material and is the basis of living cells. Your muscles, skin, hair, nails, eyes, brain, and organs are comprised of protein. In addition, antibodies, which are our body's defense mechanisms and protect us against infection, are protein. Protein is the key to both the repair of muscle tissue and growth. When we lift weights rigorously, we are breaking down muscle tissue, which is called *catabolism*. The growth and repair of the muscle tissue is called *anabolism*. Anabolism must exceed catabolism to build bigger and stronger muscles.

Sources of protein are eggs, milk and dairy products, meat and fish, beans and nuts. Sources such as eggs, milk, and fish are complete proteins; that is, they contain all the eight essential amino acids (the building blocks of protein) that are not manufactured in the human body (the other fourteen amino acids are made in the body). Therefore, the essential eight must be supplied in our food. These essential amino acids are: tryptophane, lysine, methionine, phenylalanine, threonine, valine, leucine, and isoleucine.

There are many differences of opinion as to how much protein a person needs a day. The National Research Council recommends 0.42 grams per pound of body weight. Others, particularly body builders, recommend much higher amounts due to the fact more protein is needed for both muscle repair and muscle growth for weight lifters. More protein, which makes up muscles, would necessarily be needed by the body builder to obtain the bigger muscles he wants. For those of you who are just getting into weight lifting or just trying to stay toned up I think 0.5 grams of protein per body weight is sufficient. A little excess protein won't hurt you. You will just excrete out what your body doesn't need.

The following is a basic chart for protein counting:

Food	Serving	Protein Gram Count
eggs	1	6 grams
milk	8 oz.	8 grams
cheese	1 oz.	4 grams
beans	½ cup	6-9 grams
cottage cheese	1 oz.	4 grams
yogurt	8 oz.	8 grams
liver	3 oz.	24 grams
tuna fish	3 oz.	24 grams
chicken	3 oz.	24 grams
steak	3 oz.	23 grams
ham	3 oz.	15 grams
pork chops	3 oz.	15 grams
brewer's yeast	1 oz.	12 grams
wheat germ	1 oz.	8 grams

Obviously, some meats have a higher protein count and are better for you, such as liver. Although it might taste bad to some of you, it is tremendously rich in protein, minerals, and vitamins.

Cholesterol is another touchy subject these days. For years we have heard that it is a contributing factor in arteriosclerosis and heart disease, and our intake of it after the age of thirty should be either eliminated or significantly reduced. Recent studies have now questioned whether this is true. In fact a new study has shown that a lack of cholesterol can contribute to cancer. The long and short of this is that you should consult with your doctor, be tuned in for new scientific truths, not just theories, and use lots of common sense. Don't completely cut out cholesterol but limit it sensibly by cutting down on unnecessary fats that are high in cholesterol, such as salad dressings, olive oil, and mayonnaise. The reason I am jumping the gun a bit in discussing cholesterol, which is found in fats, is because eggs are on my protein chart and are recommended. Eggs are one of nature's best foods and are a valuable source of protein and contain vitamins A, B, and D, in addition to important unsaturated fats. Although eggs contain cholesterol, they also contain lecithin, which is a homogenizing agent and breaks down fat and cholesterol into minuscule particles, which can pass readily into the tissue. Probably the best way to handle the egg question is, if you are overweight or have heart problems, consult your physician about the use of them. For the rest of you, twelve eggs a week shouldn't hurt you but help supply you with needed protein as well as vitamins and minerals. As far as milk is concerned I would follow the same precautions if you are overweight or experiencing heart trouble. For the rest of you, eight to sixteen ounces of low-fat or skim milk per day would be a good boost to your diet.

Fats

Fats are necessary for the maintenance of good health. Fat forms part of every cell, permits important intestinal bacteria to multiply, forms sex and adrenal hormones, helps regulate water balance, transports vitamins A, D, E, and K to the cells, and acts as a homogenizing agent that allows minuscule particles of fat and cholesterol to pass readily into the tissues. The foods that are high in essential fatty acids are French dressing, salad oil, cottonseed oil, avocados, nuts, and mayonnaise. If you have a deficiency in fatty acids, you might have bloatedness, fatigue, loss of sex interest, sterility, or be overweight or underweight. So do not be scared off by the word *fat* because it is a rich energy source that will supply your body with valuable nutrients. Remember my previous warnings about unnecessary cholesterol in oils, salad dressing and mayonnaise, especially if you are overweight, on a diet, or have heart problems. Although I have listed the symptoms of a deficiency in fatty acids, the vast majority of people don't have to worry about getting enough fatty acids in their diet. Their main problem is to minimize their fat intake.

Carbohydrates

Carbohydrates are best obtained mostly through fruits and vegetables, not through concentrated calories like cake, cookies, candy, and other junk food. One carbohydrate food that often gets a bad reputation is pasta. Pasta is made from flour, eggs, and water or just flour and water. The best kind of pasta to get is enriched pasta and spinach pasta. A small serving of spaghetti is only 155 calories with five grams of protein and thirty-two grams of carbohydrates. This pasta can provide you with stored-up energy. Long-distance runners often pack the carbohydrates in with lots of enriched pasta six hours or so before a race. Where you get into trouble with pasta is in the sauce, which has anywhere from 100 to another 350 calories or more if you pile it on. That marinara, ragu, or meat sauce might taste great, but it has a lot of wasted calories. If you are going to have some pasta and can't stand it plain, try to add just a small amount of a tomato sauce, not a meat sauce, or try a clam sauce for a change. Being an Italian-American, I can only go so long without some pasta, but I try to keep the sauce down and never meat sauce.

Carbohydrates, when ingested, break down quickly into glucose, which is a simple sugar used as a supply of energy. You generally need one-half gram of carbohydrates for each pound of body weight, but pick your carbs from food sources that also supply lots of protein, minerals, and vitamins (such as cottage cheese, yogurt, or enriched pasta). Bodybuilders and many dieters go on a zero or low-carbohydrate diet for a cycle. Bodybuilders do it to get cut up (become defined). However, most realize that you need some carbohydrates to keep your energy level up. If you are interested in counting your calories and carbohydrates, I recommend Barbara Kraus's *Calories and Carbohydrates*.

Water and Fiber

Water is important to the athlete because our muscles and bodies are comprised mostly of water. It is best to drink spring water that has not had additives and is rich in natural minerals. Drinking lots of water also flushes out your system of the poisons in certain foods. Water is needed in perspiration so that the body may cleanse itself from within. You have heard the expression, "I need to sweat out what I drank last night." Well, it is very true.

Fiber, nature's laxative, is the nondigestible part of food found in whole grains, nuts, fresh fruits, and vegetables. It is a necessary part of your diet. It is interesting to note that digestive problems do not occur, to a large extent, in civilizations that stick to high-fiber diets.

Vitamins

Vitamins are necessary for good health, and the athlete needs more than the average person. The athlete is constantly tearing down and building up his body, making great demands of it. His body stores of vital nutrients are being constantly depleted through his great amount of physical exercise. If his body is not supplied with the needed vitamins his energy load will decrease and injuries may result. Because so much of our food has the majority of vitamins and minerals boiled or fried out, especially at institutions, I recommend supplements. Some doctors feel this is a waste of money, but they do not take into account the lack of balanced meals most of us have, the loss of vitamins and minerals through processing, nor the added demands on the athlete's body. If you prepare your own food, try steaming instead of boiling, baking in favor of frying, and eat raw fruits and vegetables rather than always cooking them.

The following is a list of vitamins and minerals and the recommended dosages:

Vitamin A	necessary for eyesight as well as for normal cell growth, healthy skin, and skeletal development. It is found in green vegetables, carrots, apricots, yams, liver, fish, liver oils, egg yolks, butter, and cream. *Recommended dosage: 10,000 total units daily*, taken in small amounts twice or three times a day.
B complexes	important as a whole for energy production, to combat stress, hair and skin maintenance, digestive juice secretions, for blood vessels and eye maintenance. A breakdown of the B's follows:
Vitamin B1	(thiamin) necessary for preventing fatigue and helps to change glucose into energy or fat. Wheat germ is the best source and rice polish is second best. It is found in cereal grains, dry beans, peas, nuts, kidneys, heart, soybeans, and lentils. *Recommended dosage: 50 mgs.*
Vitamin B2	(riboflavin) necessary for oxygen exchange in the soft tissues and the effective use of sugar and starch. A deficiency will cause mouth irritation, dermatitis, and an abnormal intolerance to light. It is found in liver, yeast, milk, spinach, lettuce and kale. *Recommended dosage: 50 mgs.*
Vitamin B3	(niacin) helps to eliminate mental depression and is an essential part of the enzyme system. It is found in liver, yeast, wheat germ, and kidney. *Recommended dosage: 50 mgs.*
Vitamin B6	necessary for the functioning of the central nervous system as well as protein, fat, and sugar metabolism (you can see this is crucial for athletes in order to utilize protein). A deficiency will lead to loss of appetite, diarrhea, skin and mouth disorders and in the extreme, possible blindness. It is found in

brewer's yeast, whole grains, milk, egg yolks, organ meat, cabbage, and beets. This vitamin seems to be greatly in vogue now.
Recommended dosage: 100 mgs.

Vitamin B12   necessary for the functioning of the central nervous system, as well as protein, fat, and sugar metabolism. This is thought to be, by some, the most vital of the B's. A deficiency will lead to loss of appetite, decreased energy, diarrhea, skin and mouth disorder. It is found in brewer's yeast, liver, milk products, and lean meat.
Recommended dosage: 100 mgs.

choline   a vitamin B complex that is important to fat metabolism and the proper functioning of the nervous system. It is found in liver, kidneys, egg yolks, and whole grains.
Recommended dosage: 50 mgs.

inositol   another antistress vitamin that is also important for hair growth, vision, your heart's action, and digestion. It is found in liver, yeast, wheat germ, whole wheat bread, oatmeal, unrefined molasses, and corn.
Recommended dosage: 50 mgs.

pantothenic acid   a B complex vitamin that is necessary for keeping the adrenal glands working and combating stress. It is found in egg yolks, whole grains, cabbage, organ meats, and broccoli.
Recommended dosage: 50 mgs.

folic acid (Vitamin Bc)   a B complex that is essential for growth. It is necessary for the proper division of body cells and the production of RNA and DNA; also needed for production of enzymes that assimilate amino acids and is used in conversion of sugar into energy. It is found in brewer's yeast, soy flour, and kidneys.
Recommended dosage: 30 mgs.

biotin   a B complex vitamin that promotes growth. It is found in liver, kidneys, dried beans, cauliflower, chicken, whole eggs, hazel nuts, mushrooms, peas, peanuts, and bacon.
Recommended dosage: 50 mgs.

PABA	a B complex which plays an important part in hair color (some say it prevents graying) and helps to prevent sunburn. *Recommended dosage: 30 mgs.*
Vitamin B15	(pangamic acid or calcium pangmate) not recognized as a vitamin by the FDA; it is treated as a food supplement. It is used by many Russian athletes and is *purported* to be effective in treating circulatory disorders, premature aging, and heart disease. It is found in whole grains, liver, brewer's yeast, and sunflower seeds. *Recommended dosage: 50 mgs. (if you try it all at your own risk)*
Vitamin C	(ascorbic acid) one of the most important vitamins. It aids in the formation of collage, a substance that holds all cells together. It also builds up the resistance to shock and infection. A deficiency causes scurvy, bleeding gums, bruises, and the slow healing of wounds. Dr. Linus Pauling claims megadoses of C help prevent colds. *Recommended dosage: 1,000 mgs.*
Vitamin D	necessary for growth of bones and teeth, prevents fatigue andd helps burn sugar effectively. It is found in beef and chicken liver, fortified milk, egg yolks, butter, and fish oils. *Recommended dosage undetermined.*
Vitamin E	one of the most talked about and expounded, not because of its primary job, which is to supply oxygen to the cells, but because it is supposed to improve one's sexual prowess and retard the aging process. It is stored mainly in the pituitary, adrenal, and sex glands. A deficiency leads to anemia. I highly recommend this for weight lifters in dosages of *400 IUs.*

Minerals

Humans also require the following minerals: calcium, phosphorous, magnesium, sodium, potassium, sulfur, chlorine, iron, copper, cobalt, iodine, manganese, zinc, and fluorine in their daily diet. Because these minerals are found in most foods and a deficiency in them is not as likely as a vitamin deficiency, I will not chart them as completely as the vitamins, but briefly describe them in this section.

These minerals are interrelated in the synthesis of hemoglobin and the formation of red blood cells. They are crucial in nerve cell functions and body fluid maintenance. When you sweat, it is not just water, but sodium, potassium, chlorine, and phosphorous that are coming out of your system. Calcium is crucial for growth and prevention of cramping. Dairy products, nuts, and milk are the best source of calcium. Phosphorous is found in most foods. Magnesium, which is involved in the nervous system, is found in brown rice, pecans, oatmeal, hazel nuts, walnuts, corn, peanuts, brazil nuts, soya flour, barley and whole wheat. Potassium, sodium and chlorine are critical for the control and regulation of glandular secretions.

Remember, your sweat is not just water. Based on this premise, a number of companies have come out with drinks to replace your lost minerals (also called electrolytes). There is some question whether they are of much use other than quenching thirst and replacing lost fluids. The aforementioned minerals and the trace minerals zinc, cobalt, iron, iodine and manganese can be found in your protein-rich foods. I recommend a multi-mineral supplement each day to supply those which your diet might have missed. Of essential importance is potassium. A few years ago a number of people died from a potassium deficiency when they went on a liquid protein diet. If you go on a diet, make sure you get plenty of potassium from tomatoes, bananas, or a potassium supplement.

Diet

Have you noticed that even if you aren't eating any more than you did ten or twenty years ago, you now have developed a paunch, your chest might be sagging, and your butt seems to have grown? Have you been wondering how those extra beers or late-night pizza mysteriously appear at your expanded waistline or as jowls? When you get older, your metabolism slows down as well as your testosterone level. That in addition to a reduced level of activity turns into unwanted inches on your waistline, a bigger butt, and perhaps jowls. The average American gains one pound a year after the age of twenty five. One reason exercise is so important in conjunction with dieting is that it helps to burn up calories. But more important if you diet without exercise you lose some fat but other fat replaces muscle. You will lose weight without the exercise but you will have a higher body-fat content, less muscles and look bad. Just because over one-third of all Americans and the majority of Americans over thirty five are overweight doesn't mean that you have to carry unwanted pounds or inches. Although it might be a little harder to get in shape and tone up your body when you are over thirty five, it doesn't mean you should be discouraged or not even try.

Should you go on a weight-loss diet at the same time you are working out or should you try to lose your excess weight first? I think that exercise can help you in your weight-loss program, provided you take care to eat enough complex carbohydrates to provide glucose for energy needed for strenuous exercise.

In the 1960s and 50s, people who were reducing were most likely on a low-calorie diet. This was based on the fact that you lose weight when you burn up more calories than you take in. Each pound accounts for 3,500 calories, and people were on diets consisting of 1,000 to 2,000 calories a day. Later, low-carbohydrate diets became the craze, popularized by *Dr. Atkin's Diet Revolution.* It seemed like everyone who was on a diet was counting carbs and losing up to ten or fourteen pounds in the first two weeks. A criticism of this low-carb diet is that the initial loss is due to a loss of fluids. Every gram of carbohydrate in our body can hold four grams of water. Therefore, when you greatly cut back on the carbs, your body can't store as much water and you lose weight. Another criticism of the low-carb diet is that it causes you to have a significant energy loss because of the low blood-sugar levels (remember carbohydrates are transformed into glucose, a simple sugar that gives you energy). This in turn reflects on your athletic performance as well as your irritability.

In the 1970s the country embraced Dr. Tarnover's *The Scarsdale Medical Diet.* His objective was to devise a diet that offered rapid weight loss as well as being nutritionally balanced. In addition the SMD allows for a lifetime keep-trim weight-control program. The SMD is a weight-loss program for adults with no medical or dietary restrictions and after a doctor's approval. This diet is generally referred to as a high-protein low-calorie diet. On his diet, there are no vitamin or mineral deficiencies. On the SMD, you average 1,000 calories per day, which is broken up nutritionally into 43 percent protein, 22.5 percent fat and 34.5 percent carbohydrates. Protein is supplied in meat, fish, poultry, protein bread, and cheese. You will note that carbohydrates are cut back but included in protein bread, fruits, and vegetables. Fat consumption is cut down significantly, so the body then uses up the fats stored already in the body in the form of excess weight. Limiting the fat intake explains why the SMD weight loss is so significant. When the body burns more fat than it normally does, an excess of ketones are produced. Ketones are partially metabolized products of fat, which are eliminated through the urine. When carbohydrates and fats are limited in intake and do not meet the body's caloric needs, your system draws upon stored fat. Ketones are the result of your body's metabolism burning off this excess fat. Ketone's also help curb one's appetite. SMD states that although this diet's combination of foods increases fat metabolism and ketone production, they are not raised to an unhealthy level. In SMD, Tarnover recommends following the diet for two weeks, then go on the keep-trim diet. The Keep-Trim diet supposedly will stabilize the weight loss achieved on the SMD. If you want to lose more weight on this plan you go on and off the SMD every two weeks till you obtain the weight you desire. The on and off program is said to be psychological. You won't be as tempted if you know you are going off soon.

Criticism, including mine, of this diet is that the greatly reduced carbohydrates will make you irritable and cause a loss of energy. There is also a significant amount of criticism that the diet is too high in protein. Your body can only use so much protein, and to use protein as a source of energy is the most inefficient use of it. I think that cutting down on dairy products from your diet deprives your body of a valuable source of protein, vitamins, and minerals. Also on his "don't list" are potatoes and rice. Potatoes are a valuable carbohydrate containing protein, vitamins, and minerals, and as long as you don't use butter or sour cream, it doesn't contain many calories. Rice, especially brown rice, is loaded with nutrients and along with potatoes (never fried or with oil) are a good source of energy. He allows you all lean meats, yet ham and all pork products (he doesn't allow sausage) have the highest fat and lowest protein count of any meat. The SMD doesn't distinguish between the vegetables that are high in calories, such as lima beans and corn and low-calorie ones like broccoli and radishes. The same distinction is lacking in his fruits. An apple is far more fattening than a grapefruit (although he always starts his breakfasts off with a half a grapefruit) or strawberries. However, his books have a lot of very valid points and were effective in achieving weight loss for numerous people. His variety of diets—the international, the gourmet, the money saver, and the vegetarian diet—offers a wide and interesting choice.

For those of you that are healthy with no restrictions from your doctor I would recommend first simple rules to lose weight that almost everyone can use. Then I will give you a low-fat low-calorie diet that will be very effective. The reason for the low-fat diet is that fats have twice as many calories per gram as protein or carbohydrates (fats have nine calories per gram while carbs and protein have only four). Although fats are essential to your diet, you only need 10 percent of your diet to consist of fats or ten to twenty grams of fat per day. That's not hard to do because even chicken breasts which I highly recommend (with the skin taken off) have some fat in them.

Low Fat Dieting Rules

1. Limit yourself to no more than two light beers or two glasses of dry wine or two ounces of vodka mixed with grapefruit juice, cranberry juice, or club soda. You may mix so you can have one light beer and one vodka each day. But avoid those mixers like tonic water, orange juice, or soda.

2. Cut out all junk food, i.e., cake, cookies, pastry, doughnuts, candy, ice cream, soda, etc.

3. Don't overeat! You don't need to have second helpings. Fortunately, you all don't have Italian or Jewish mothers pushing food at you and not happy with you till you have eaten everything on the table as well as in the refrigerator.

4. Avoid excess salt and dietetic foods and drinks because the sodium causes your body to retain excess water.

5. In this day and age, it is not impolite to refuse a fattening desert at a dinner party.

6. Try to have only one dinner of lean meat a week. The rest of your dinners should be mostly broiled or baked fish and some dinners of turkey or chicken without the skin. This change in your diet will alone cause you to lose excess weight in surprising amounts.

7. When you have enriched pasta, try not to have any sauce, but if you must, use only a little tomato sauce.

8. Never eat any fried foods, especially chicken or potatoes.

9. Don't butter your bread or use butter or sour cream on your potato.

10. Don't use oil or regular salad dressings on your salad. Try to stick to vinegar or lemon juice on your salad. If you have to, use low-calarie dressings but never any with oil, sour cream, cheese, or cream. Avoid mayonnaise at all times.

11. Try to limit your fruits to low-calorie ones like grapefruit, strawberries, cantaloupe, pineapples, honeydew melons, and cherries.

12. Try to limit your vegetables to lower calorie ones like broccoli, chick peas, string beans, eggplant, asparagus, cucumbers, lettuce, cabbage, celery, radishes, peppers, onions, mushrooms, spinach, tomatoes, and squash. Avoid those fattening vegetables like corn, lima beans, peas, and carrots. Peas and carrots, if used, should be in very small amounts.

13. Avoid all sauces on your food except lemon or vinegar based.

14. Eat slowly, and chew your food thoroughly.

15. Try to eat a king's breakfast, a prince's lunch and a pauper's dinner. It is better for your digestion. Remember, at your breakfast, don't use any pork products, hash browns, fried potatoes, pancakes, or waffles. However, you can feast on a gourmet's breakfast consisting of eggs or omelettes in any form provided that fat is eliminated (or almost eliminated) in the preparation. Whole wheat toast is okay and so is French toast made with whole wheat bread and eggs. Instead of syrup, try nonsweetened applesauce.

The enclosed diet is my variation of a daily foot allotment given out to heart patients. As you can see, it has variations from 1,000 to 2,000 calories per day.

Modified Doctor's Heart-Patient Diet

This diet is planned to meet your specific nutritional needs. Your doctor has indicated the meal plan that provides you with the appropriate number of calories each day in a balanced nutritional intake. This specified caloric level is met by consuming the required number of servings in each food group as indicated in your daily food allowance.

Foods are divided into six groups called exchange lists. Portions of all foods within an exchange list have approximately equal carbohydrate and caloric values. By selecting different foods within each of the six exchange lists you can add variety to your meals. If, for example, you are to follow the 1,600 calorie diet, your lunch would be: 1 choice (or serving) from each of the fruit, fat, and bread exchange lists, 1 serving from the vegetable A exchange list, 2 servings from the meat exchange list (for example, 2 oz. meat or 1 oz. meat and 1 egg), and coffee or tea.

Important: It is important that you eat the amounts and kinds of food indicated in your Daily Food Allowance. The nutritive value of your meals and nourishments has been arranged to provide you with balanced nutrition throughout the day.

Measuring food: Portion sizes must be accurate; weigh or measure when necessary. For this you will need measuring spoons and a standard 8-oz. measuring cup. All measurements are **level.** Cooked foods are measured **after** cooking. The use of a small scale to determine portion sizes is helpful until you are familiar with the appearance of the correct serving size.

Food preparation: Meats may be baked, boiled, or broiled. Your foods may be prepared with the family meals, but be sure your portion is removed before any extra fat or flour is added. Fried foods should be eaten only if an allowed fat choice is used for frying. Combination dishes such as stews and casseroles may be eaten if permitted ingredients are used in the amounts specified in your Daily Food Allowance.

Avoid these foods: Sugar, candy, honey, jam, jelly, preserves, marmalade, syrup, pies, cakes and cookies not listed in the bread exchange list, pastries, condensed milk, sweetened carbonated beverages, chewing gums containing sugar, fried, scalloped and creamed foods, beer, wine and other alcoholic beverages and snack items such as pretzels, popcorn, and potato chips.

Instructions: Follow the Daily Food Allowance for your specific calorie level, freely selecting from the food groups on the next page. Follow exactly the portions as indicated for each meal. Do not omit any of the foods indicated in the Daily Food Allowance.

Daily Food Allowance

Number of servings for

	1,000 cal.	1,400 cal.	1,600 cal.	1,800 cal.	2,000 cal.
Breakfast					
fruit	1	1	1	1	1
meat	1	1	1	1	1
bread	½	1	2	1	2
fat	–	1	2	2	2
coffee or tea (as desired)					
Lunch					
meat	2	2	2	2	3
vegetable list A	1	1	1	1	1
bread	–	1	1	1	1
fat	–	1	1	1	1
fruit	1	1	1	1	1
coffee or tea (as desired)					
Dinner					
meat	3	3	3	3	4
vegetable list A	1	1	1	1	1
vegetable list B	1	1	1	1	1
bread	–	1	1	1	1
fat	–	1	1	1	1
fruit	1	1	1	1	1
coffee or tea (as desired)					

Evening   yogurt with wheat germ or milk-and-egg protein drink with 8 oz. of skim milk

Food Groups

Vegetable A Exchange

Amount per serving: raw—
   any amount cooked—1 cup

asparagus	lettuce
broccoli	mushrooms
Brussels sprout	okra
cabbage	peppers
cauliflower	radishes
celery	sauerkraut
cucumbers	spinach
eggplant	summer squash
green beans	tomatoes*
greens	wax beans

* Limit to one tomato or ½ cup
tomato juice per serving

Fruit Exchange

fresh, frozen, or canned
   without sugar

	Serving
apricots	2 medium
apricot nectar	½ cup
banana	½ small
blackberries	1 cup
blueberries	⅔ cup
cantaloupe (6″ diam.)	¼
cherries	10 large
dates	2
grapefruit	½ small
grapefruit juice	½ cup
grape juice	¼ cup
honeydew melon	1″ slice
nectarine	1 medium

Bread Exchange

	Serving
bread	1 slice
biscuit	1
crackers, saltine	5
graham	2
round thin	6
muffin, plain	1
cereal, cooked	½ cup
cereal, dry (not (not pre-sweetened)	¾ cup
potatoes, white	½ cup
rice (cooked), pre-ferably brown	½ cup
spaghetti noodles (cooked)	½ cup
macaroni (cooked)	½ cup
egg noodles (cooked)	½ cup
corn	⅓ cup

Meat Exchange

Baked, boiled, or
broiled

	Serving
Meat (no pork pro-ducts), poultry, fish	
luncheon meats	
oysters, clams, shrimp	5 small
tuna, salmon (water pack	¼ cup
egg	1
cheese	1 oz.
cottage cheese	¼ cup
peanut butter	1 tablespoon

Fruit Exchange (continued)

peach	1 medium
pear	1 small
pineapple	½ cup
pineapple juice	⅓ cup
prunes, dried	2 medium
prune juice	¼ cup
raisins	2 tablespoons
raspberries	1 cup
strawberries	1 cup
tangerine	1 large

Fat Exchange

	Serving
butter/margarine	1 teaspoon
light cream	2 tablespoons
French dressing	1 tablespoon
cream cheese	1 tablespoon
olives	5
nuts	6 small
avocado	½" slice

Allowed as desired

Foods

artificially sweetened beverages or
soda pop containing less than 10 calories
per can, coffee or tea (no sugar or
cream), fat-free broth or bouillon,
rhubarb or cranberries (no sugar added),
sour or dill pickles, unflavored gelatin

Seasonings
herbs, spices, salt, mustard, lemon,
flavor extracts, calorie-free sugar
substitutes, vinegar

Supplements

If you have three balanced meals a day, you should not need supplements. However, most of us don't eat the balanced meals we should or are eating in restaurants or institutions, where many of the vitamins and minerals are taken out. That is why I recommend vitamin and mineral supplements. When I was coaching at Notre Dame and even at the Denver Broncos, we regularly handed out protein supplements to our players, preferably a milk-and-egg protein supplement. We wanted to be sure that our men got all the protein they needed. If you are a middle-aged executive just toning up and you aren't missing meals, then you probably don't need a protein supplement. However, if you have to miss meals or are more serious in your bodybuilding program, you may want to take two ounces of a good milk-and-egg protein supplement with eight ounces of skim milk or papaya juice daily. Make sure you count the extra calories in the protein supplement.

Steroids

Steroids are the last subject in this chapter because I want my comments on this chapter to remain fresh in your mind. Although a significant number of bodybuilders and a number of other athletes have used them, I am definitely opposed to them. Not just because they are not natural or because you shrink quickly after usage is stopped. The dangerous side effects that might occur are liver or kidney damage, impotency, skin problems or loss of hair. Since they have not been around long, there has not been time enough to check for possible damages to human chromosomes. The children of those who took steroids might be born with birth defects. The 1980s will bring a lot of answers to many questions about the dangers of steroids.

In summary, I always recommend that my trainees avoid steroids as well as any other drugs.

AEROBICS

Aerobic exercising refers to various exercises that stimulate both heart and lung activity long enough for beneficial changes to occur. These exercises involve the maximum intake and utilization of air (aerobics meaning *air*) and result in an increased lung capacity. The heart becomes a more effective pump, and respiratory muscles also increase in strength and endurance. As a result, there is a greater intake and diffusion of oxygen to the blood. The increased aerobic capacity leads to greater endurance. The relationship between aerobic capacity and physical well being is simple and direct. In addition to increasing the body's capacity for utilizing oxygen and promoting a healthier cardiovascular system, aerobic exercising has been effective in combating injuries to the body and producing a higher level of mental alertness.

The first thirty seconds to one minute of exertion are anaerobic (without oxygen)—the body does not need oxygen to reach the muscles for a response. This explains how we react immediately to an instinctual response. However, once this response is over, the muscles must have oxygen to perform. (This is what *most* weight training is, although circuit training can be aerobic.) The goals of aerobic exercising are to increase performance and endurance and to adapt the body's support system (bones, muscles, joints, etc.) to accommodate the increased physical activity. Exercises designed to improve aerobic capacity must be of a dynamic nature, involving at least one-sixth of all the body's muscles. The only way to improve or maintain one's endurance is to train. Training is measured doses of overexertion. The heart must be placed under long-term, sustained physical activity. The cardiovascular system consists of the heart and the lungs. The heart is a four chambered muscle about the size of a man's fist. It lies a little to the left of the center of your chest. The heart pumps blood, which carries oxygen to all parts of the body.

As we exercise more, we increase the need for oxygen to be delivered to our muscles. Training will increase the heart's efficiency, making it stronger and thereby increasing its pumping capacity.

Heart disease is the leading killer in our nation today, with almost 1 million Americans dying from heart-related problems each year. One in three adults suffers from cardiac-circulatory ailments. Aerobic exercising is ideal for preventive measures in conditioning the body against a heart attack and can also have a restorative effect on an impaired circulation. Exercise is a most effective medicine, precautionary or recuperative, for your heart. As your respiratory muscles strengthen, they reduce their resistance to air flow, allowing greater amounts of air into the lungs. The more oxygen you take in the more the blood is pumped. The heart, like any muscle, can be strengthened. A strong heart pumps more blood with each beat, reducing the amounts of strokes per minute. An increased aerobic capacity causes the heart to strain less, in turn reducing blood pressure and the amount of work the heart has to do. Muscle tone is also increased with a greater aerobic endurance, allowing better circulation. Finally, aerobic conditioning increases the amount of red-blood cells and hemoglobin in the blood. Hemoglobin is the part of the blood that carries oxygen. An increased number of hemoglobin, therefore, makes the blood a more efficient oxygen carrier.

I recommend a complete physical examination and electrocardiogram (EKG) before undertaking an aerobic exercise program. The EKG should be taken while you are exercising, such as on a treadmill or on a stationary bicycle. The EKG and examination should determine any existing heart or health problems that would dictate adjusting your exercise program accordingly. The only restriction age places on the amount of exercise is how long it will take you to condition. If you have been inactive for many years, you should be less vigorous in your approach and proceed at a slower rate. Such conditions as obesity, diabetes, and chronic and congenital heart problems may prohibit certain exercises such as running and jogging, but it is possible to achieve aerobic conditioning through walking or some other less strenuous exercise.

The benefits of each exercise depends on the duration and intensity involved. The minimum program for fitness is three thirty-minute exercises per week. If you jog five miles per hour, you must walk twice as long to burn the same amount of calories and earn the same aerobic value. If you cycle at ten mph, you burn the same amount of calories as jogging at five mph. To measure the aerobic intensity of each exercise, use the number of heart beats per minute (pulse rate) to see if the physical activity is sufficient enough to produce the desired training effect. To calculate your pulse rate, place your thumb on the right or left side of your neck. Keeping time with a watch with a second hand, count the beats for ten seconds. Then multiply the amount by six. The intensity of the exercise should raise the pulse by 60 percent. The minimum heart rate for a training effect should be 170 minus your age; this would be ascertained a few moments after you have completed your exercising. The heart rate should not exceed 220 minus your age, or you have overtaxed your heart and must proceed slower.

In his book, *The New Aerobics,* Doctor Kenneth H. Cooper (M. Evans, 1970) uses a point system in addition to the increased pulse rate to determine the effectiveness of each exercise. The more energy that is expended with each exercise, the more points you receive. Following Cooper's point chart program, the exercises become progressively more intense, though not necessarily in amount but in the intensity in which they are performed. For example, if you are on a running program at two miles three times a week, the distance would not have to change, but your time should decrease with each succeeding week to get the benefits of aerobic conditioning. More points are allotted in accordance with the intensity of the exercise, with the goal being thirty points per week—Cooper's minimum standard of fitness. My criticism of the point system as established by Cooper is that he does not in fact award equal points for energy expended, being somewhat low for some athletic activities such as lacrosse or rugby. Also, it should be recognized that twenty minutes of effort is not four times as effective as five minutes, nor are four sessions per week as effective as two.

The benefits of aerobic conditioning, then, are many. A healthier cardiovascular system aids in preventing and recuperating from a heart attack, tension is reduced, and you feel more invigorated and alert. Some diabetics on an aerobics program have found that the exercises help improve the body's capability to process sugar and reduces their insulin intake. It is important to remember that, in undertaking an aerobics-exercise program, you do not strain yourself to the point of exhaustion in the beginning. This defeats the purpose of the program, leaving you fatigued. It is also important that you exercise regularly to build up your aerobic capacity. Exercising at the same time each day can help you get into a habit of exercising. And exercising with a group may help you in your determination to reach your aerobic capacity.

Circuit Weight Training

Circuit weight training usually comprises multistations of weight-training equipment, either Nautilus, Universal, Paramount, free-weights, or some other combination of equipment. When I was coaching full time, I only employed circuit training for maintenance programs and for the logistics advantages (you can push a lot of people through in a short amount of time). I generally don't like circuit training for body building because I believe you get a lot more out of the exercises when you do them by body part together (e.g., do all your bench presses together before you go on to your chin ups or military presses). By working all the exercises for that body part together before going on to another body-part exercise, you get far better development of that body part.

However, the advantages of circuit training are that you get better cardiovascular conditioning than if you worked a regular weight-training program, and you do get some body-toning effects. I do believe that is not nearly as good a conditioner as running, swimming, or bicycling. In the usual Nautilus circuit, you start with the largest muscles groups first—the hip-and-back machine, then either the leg extension, leg curl, and leg press or the combination leg-extension/leg-press machine, then the chest machine, which combines a seated upright bench press with an incline fly to work all parts of your chest. Resting only thirty seconds between each machine, not between each part of the compound machines, you then proceed to either the Nautilus lat pulldown or combination back machine, which has a pullover mechanism and a frontal lat pulldown. From there you go on to the double-shoulder machine, which works all heads of your deltoids, or the trap machine if your club has it first. Then you proceed to the double-arm machine, which comprises the curling machine for your biceps and tricep extension for your triceps or back of your arms. Nautilus recommends one set for twelve reps to failure on each machine. As you will note in my description of their equipment, they advise you to be smooth in your motions and return to the starting position slowly. By returning to the starting position slowly, you are utilizing the negative aspect of the exercise also. The negative aspect of each exercise is important also. Remember the positive aspect is when you lift the weight such as in the press, and the negative aspect is when you let the weight down.

In the Universal circuit, you usually start with the leg extension for eight to twelve reps then roll over and do the leg curl for the same amount of reps (you should only be able to do two-thirds the amount of weight you can do on the leg extension), then the leg press for eight to twelve reps. Don't do full extensions on the leg press if you have any knee problems. The next station is the sit-up board, then the bench press, the chin-up bars, the military press, the low pulley for curls or cable rowing, and lastly the lat pulldown. If you use the Universal or Paramount circuit, rest thirty seconds between each station. When you start, go through the stations for one set for the first week, then two sets three times a week the second week. The third week try three sets of each circuit three times a week. That should tone you up and help to get you in condition. One advantage to the Paramount equipment is that there are dual stacks, so that you work each arm independently as well as each leg. Therefore, if one arm or leg is stronger than another, you will get equal development, and the stronger one won't take up the slack.

You don't need the aforementioned equipment but can set up a circuit with free weights or a combination of free weights and machines as I did at Notre Dame. A typical circuit like this would have a quad-ham machine first, then a squat rack (preferably a power rack with pins, which is safer than two bare racks), a bench press, an incline press, a chin-up bar or lat pulldown, a rack with a bar or dumbbells to do military presses with, then an easy-curl bar or dumbbells to curl with and a bench with another easy-curl bar to do lying tricep extensions for the back of your arms. Either before this equipment or after, you could put a sit-up board (or a sit-up board first and a Roman chair last).

However, whichever circuit you use you should make sure you stretch out first and warm up before starting. Make sure you don't take more than thirty seconds between each set, or you won't get the aerobic effect of circuit training.

Running

Running/jogging is one of the most effective aerobic exercises. Muscle tone and strength increase, and running promotes better circulation. It does not demand a great deal of time and the benefits derived are not affected by traffic or weather. And, outside of buying equipment, it costs relatively little. The most visible benefit of running is the weight loss. Walking at one mph burns off 135 calories per hour, and walking at four mph can burn off 400 calories. Jogging at five mph equals 550 calories. Running at five and one-half mph will use up 630 calories and at a seven mph pace will burn up 750 calories. Running also aids in supressing the appetite. Blood is taken away from the stomach and used on the muscles involved while running. However, a rapid weight loss may also be a sign of overexertion.

Besides the high caloric ultilization running gives, there are significant cardiovascular benefits. The number of red-blood cells increase, breathing becomes deeper, and the hemoglobin in the blood becomes more acidic, making the red-blood cells attract oxygen more readily. As the lungs gain in their oxygen consumption, the heart strengthens and in turn reduces the blood pressure.

In addition to acting as a safeguard against heart attack, it has been speculated that running promotes mental health—combating depression, reducing anxiety, and changing self-destructive patterns such as smoking and drinking. Theoretically, as your body strengthens, so does your mind. Depression is manifested by both physical and emotional symptoms. Depression can be brought on physically and, therefore, being physically fit and in good health can be an effective means of combating depression. Physically fit patients also respond more readily to psychotherapy. A poor self-image can be treated with a running program with significant results. As the body becomes more conditioned and attractive, one's self-image will most likely improve. It has been speculated that running produces this emotional balance by fulfilling self-assertion needs, testing one's limits and achieving a tangible control over one's appearance. Insomnia has also been treated effectively with running. The increased exercise program produces a healthy fatigue in the body, and you sleep deeper. The subconscious is fully released in this deep sleep, and dreams can surface. Studies are now being taken on the effectiveness of a running program in treating alcoholics and people who suffer from migraine headaches.

Your form while running is most important. The heel should be the first part of the foot to touch the ground. The heel should come down as softly as possible, avoid pounding on the ground. The legs should fully extend with each stride; and the faster the pace, the longer the stride. Run with your fists lightly closed, not clenched. The arms should be flexible and the hands should not raise up much higher than the waist. Keep your eyes up, shoulders relaxed, and your posture as comfortable as possible. Avoid leaning forward too much. Establishing a rhythm to your breathing can help you set your pace.

Choosing the right equipment is essential to a running program. Inappropriate clothing can increase the likelihood of an accident. A good, well-fitting shoe is the runner's most important piece of equipment. It not only guards against injury to the knee, legs, hips, and joints, but it can also enhance performance. The running shoe's purpose is to protect the foot from the constant pounding on the pavement. A properly fitted shoe should have about one-half inch between the big toe and the front of the shoe. The foot should fit firmly into the shoe but not too snugly. It is advisable to get a half size bigger than you wear normally, since the foot swells while running. There should also be a wedge on the back of the shoe that lifts the heel up. This relieves the strain on the Achilles tendon and calf muscles. The shoe should be flexible enough to allow comfortable movement. The shoe should have a flat heel, and an inner sole to give solid support. The sole should be made of a thick, rubberized material. Ripple-type soles are best for pavement jogging, while gripper-type soles work best on a cinder track or dirt path. Those accustomed to wearing heeled shoes should walk in the flat running shoes for a while to stretch the calf muscles. Sock wear is optional, depending on the individual, though they are helpful in preventing blisters. The shirts and shorts you wear should be made of a porous, absorbent material. Clothing should also be lightweight and comfortable. Cotton is ideal, and nylon should be avoided as it holds in too much of the body heat while running. The human body adapts well to environmental conditions given the chance. You should allow a week for the body to adjust to changes in the weather or a higher altitude. The clothing you wear can help your body adjust more readily. In extreme heat, you can run shirtless, while you should wear a hat and gloves in the cold (one-half of your body heat escapes through the scalp).

There are many courses available for a running program. Grassy paths in a park are ideal since they are soft and resilient. But they are scarce and may be dangerous for night running since your limited vision may prevent you from seeing holes and bumps. A dirt path is also ideal, provided it isn't covered with stones that may hurt the feet. Avoid too soft courses, such as sand, since it can overstress the feet and legs and lead to hypertension of the joints. Most cinder and wood tracks are circular, and joggers find them to be boring and repetitive. Asphalt or concrete roads are the most accessible to runners. Though they are usually smooth, minor aches and pains may arise from the constant pounding. Adjusting your form may correct this, though most runners who use asphalt and concrete courses are prone to injuries of this nature. Changing the course or path you run on helps to avoid boredom. Try to avoid running near traffic or factories. The carbon monoxide they give off inhibits the body's capacity to carry oxygen and may cause dizziness and shortness of breath. As I mentioned before, it takes the body about a week to get used to increased temperatures. It is important to replace lost body fluids from the increased perspiration and salt loss. Fluids should be taken slowly, and salt tablets or using more table salt on your food will compensate for the salt deficit. Allow two to three hours after eating before you run and make the prerun meal light. It is preferable to run on an empty stomach entirely. With a full stomach, the blood you need to supply oxygen to the muscles is in the stomach aiding in digestion. You tire more easily without the blood and oxygen you need to fuel your muscles. Also refrain from smoking thirty minutes before and after any strenuous exercise. You inhale carbon monoxide from cigarettes, and they should be avoided as it cuts down on hemoglobin's ability to carry oxygen. Though many joggers have found running to be an impetus to quit smoking, you must have a genuine desire to stop as well.

Runners are susceptible to a variety of injuries. Preventive measures include proper warm-up and warm-down exercises, the correct form while running, and the right equipment. Improper footwear can lead to lower-leg-stress fractures. Your warm-up and warm-down exercises should include sit-ups, since running does not do much for the stomach. There are also various calisthenics that are helpful in limbering up the body before a run and warming it down afterwards. Toe touching, side stretches, and leg extensions all increase the flexibility necessary for a safe and productive run. To strengthen the calf muscles, stand with your feet parallel, toes pointed inward slightly. Raise up on your left leg, shifting your total body weight to that leg. Alternate with your right leg. Another exercise for stretching the calves is to stand straight, about three feet away from a wall. Lean forward with your palms extended into the wall, keeping your feet as flat as possible on the ground. To strengthen the ankles, hop lightly on each foot. The knees can be strengthened by dropping from a standing position, bending into a deep squat. (See the flexibility section for more exercises.)

Certain problems may be caused by improper equipment. *Runner's toe* is a hemorrhage under the toenail. This is caused by jamming the toes against the front of the shoe. Although this is not serious, it is a sign that you need a better fitting shoe. Blisters may be caused by too much friction between the skin and shoe. Powdering the foot with talcum powder and wearing a cotton sock can help relieve this problem. If you do get a blister, lance it with a sterilized needle, put a first-aid dressing on, and bandage it, making sure the area is kept clean to prevent infection. Arch pains may arise from improper shoes or a bone defect. A podiatrist may be able to rectify the problem. A podiatrist is a foot-care specialist who can fit you with a special device to correct running problems and, in extreme cases, perform corrective surgery. Hip injuries can be caused by unequal leg lengths. A lift placed in the shorter leg's shoe by a podiatrist can correct this.

Overtaxing unconditioned muscles and ligaments can result in painful injuries. Knees may become swollen with liquid due to overuse. An exercise to alleviate or prevent this is to sit on the edge of a desk and raise your leg until it is fully extended in front of you, lowering it slowly. This strengthens the quadriceps, which are the muscles in front of the thigh. Shin splints are a pain in the front portion of the lower leg and may be caused by pounding the pavement too hard. Chronic overuse of a muscle can lead to tendonitis, which is a pain and swelling of the affected area. Again, this may arise from proper footwear or lack of a warm-up and warm-down period. Resting will help relieve the pain from tendonitis. Return to running gradually. Sprains may result from a severe fall or twisting of a muscle. Ice, applied quickly, will help to limit the swelling. You should not resume running until you can walk with no pain. Taking one tablet of vitamin C for every hour you run is effective in protecting the muscles and ligaments against injury. Remember to allow yourself time to condition your muscles. Overtaxing yourself can lead to serious injury and set back any aerobic benefits you may have gained. I discourage people from starting directly on a running program unless they have been exercising regularly. Walking allows the heart to accommodate the new physical demands and lets the body's muscles and tendons adjust as well. With a doctor'a approval, a jogging program may be undertaken if the aerobic conditioning received from walking is sufficient. Remember

to work slowly into any exercise program if you have remained inactive
for many years.

Swimming

Swimming offers superior muscular and cardiovascular benefits from a
relatively small investment of time. Swimming's dynamic movement
exercises all the major muscle groups and is very good for the back and
spine. It is as efficient as running for the cardiovascular system. One mile
of swimming equals four miles of jogging in the benefits and conditioning
produced. I highly recommend swimming for those who cannot use an
aerobic running program. There is also less chance of strains and injuries
likely to occur while swimming than in most sports. A breastroke will use
up 450 calories per hour, the back stroke burns up 450 calories, and the
crawl will use up 800 calories per hour. An aerobic swimming program
should last for at least ten minutes a swim to produce the desired benefits.
As with running, increased levels of assuredness, reduced anxiety and an
improved sense of well-being have been reported with swimming.
Swimming increases the lung's capacity for holding oxygen. The added
water pressure placed on the body strengthens the oxygen intake process.
Although you cannot increase the size of your lungs, you can help them
work more efficiently. The capillaries, which are extensions of the arteries
that bring the blood from the heart, increase in number. The capillaries
are the site of oxygen pickup from the lungs and oxygen transferral to the
muscle cells in the blood. As the number of capillaries increase, the higher
and quicker the oxygen can get to the muscles involved.

With swimming becoming increasingly popular, it is no longer just a
summer sport. Most apartment complexes, municipal recreation, and
YMCA's offer swimming facilities. Heated pools help combat prevailing
weather conditions, and I strongly urge the use of an indoor, heated pool.
The body does not have to adjust to varying temperatures, and there is
less risk of accidents.

When swimming, the body should be horizontal with the head held
low. This gives the least resistance to swimming. Arms should enter and
pull the water with straight elbows. Once in the water, bend them to a
ninety-degree angle, returning to an extended position before coming up
out of the water. Hold the hands outward diagonally as it enters the
water. This cuts down on water resistance and helps propel you forward
efficiently. For your breathing, you should inhale air when you start to
bring your arm out of the water. Breathe in on the side your arm comes
up on. Breathe in with your nose and exhale through both nose and
mouth.

When buying a suit, choose a snug-fitting suit made of a lightweight, flexible material. Loose suits increase resistance to movement in water and impair your buoyancy. Heavy suits, such as cutoffs will weigh you down. Nylon is ideal since it is lightweight and stands up well to chlorine and salt water. Washing your swim suit after a swim helps to avoid discoloration. Showering after a swim with a good moisturizing soap will restore your body's natural oils. Skin and eye problems may occur from high chemical levels in a pool. *Swimmer's itch* is an allergic reaction from swimming in fresh water that contains parasites that use muskrats and certain birds as host-carriers. This can be relieved with using calamine lotion. *Swimmer's ear* is an irritation of the ear canal from a bacterial infection. It is good to get in the habit of drying the ear with rubbing alcohol after a swim. Earplugs also help prevent infections; they should be moistened so they can slip in easily. Goggles help prevent chlorine irritation in the eyes. Dipping the goggles in the pool before swimming will prevent the moisture from fogging up your vision.

Cramps occur while swimming from a muscle tightening from a lack of blood. Most pass momentarily and can be relieved by applying pressure firmly. Sprains are from overtaxing weak muscles and insufficient training. *Swimmer's shoulder* is from overuse of the overhand swing. Flexibility exercises and proper warm-up and warm-down procedures can help you to avoid these muscular problems. Jumping jacks, shoulder rolls, leg stretches, and torso twists all help stretch the muscles before a swim. To warm up before a swim, lie flat in the water, face down. Holding onto the edge of the pool, kick your feet back and forth. At the same time, turn your head sideways to breathe in and out in rhythm to your kicking.

I recommend indoor swimming since the pools are usually heated and a lifeguard is in attendance to help in the case of an accident. If you choose to swim in fresh or sea water, there are some extra precautions you should take. Do not swim immediately after a heavy meal, as the muscle cramps you may get can impair your swimming ability. Wherever you swim, make sure a lifeguard or other people are around. Although a swim in the ocean can be invigorating, there are many dangers such as sharks, jellyfish, and other sea creatures. A jellyfish sting should be attended to immediately. Rubbing wet sand on it helps relieve the pain, as will vinegar or meat tenderizer. Most beach lifeguards have the proper medication to treat such injuries. You should also be aware of the changing tides and currents when swimming in the ocean. Do not take risks and overestimate your ability to fight an undertow. Also never swim out of the range of the lifeguard.

Incidentally, swimming is just about the best therapy there is for recuperating from a knee injury. Just ask your physician.

Bicycling

Bicycling produces great overall aerobic endurance. An advantage of cycling is that it is very hard to overexert yourself. The muscles involved in cycling tire sooner than the heart. The buttocks, quadriceps, and calves are all strengthened by bicycling. A bike can also be incorporated into a daily regimen, such as cycling to work. However, cycling is dependent upon the weather and traffic, although the proper clothing can help combat the prevailing weather conditions. Bicycling also burns up a significant amount of calories. At six miles per hour, you use up 270 calories. Increasing the speed to ten mph, 400 calories are used in an hour, and 650 calories are expended from a pace of thirteen mph.

When buying a bicycle, choose a model with a light frame and large wheels. Folding bikes are impractical to ride. Changeable gears are also recommended for shifting speeds and increasing the intensity of the exercise. A tachometer will determine the revolutions per minute. And a stopwatch is helpful for calculating speed and duration. The seat should be positioned so that the leg is fully stretched to reach the pedal. When riding, the ball of the foot, not the toes or arch, should be placed on the pedal. You should pedal completely around, not allowing one foot to rest as the other leg pumps. Your posture should be comfortable, with your eyes looking straight ahead and the hands steering the handlebars. Climbing hills on a bike provides better aerobic conditioning than riding flat surfaces, as the energy expended going up an incline is greater. Hill-climbing is also great for strengthening the calf muscles.

Stationary bicycles have all the advantages and none of the disadvantages of outdoor riding. Though one may bore more easily on a stationary bike, it can offer an excellent testing or conditioning program. An ergometer on one can help determine your exercise tolerance, which is helpful in undertaking an aerobic conditioning program on a bicycle. If you choose or are restricted to a stationary bicycle, choose one with as large a flywheel as possible. Many come with speed and mileage indicators which are great aids in charting your progress. They range in price from $50 on up to $900. Also, make sure the bike you choose has brake resistance. These are also great therapy for knee injuries.

It is quite easy to keep track of your aerobic progress on a cycling exercise program. All you need is a stopwatch and tachometer feature added on to the bike. First, record your pulse rate. Starting out on your ride, proceed slowly until you reach your training pulse rate (remember the ideal is 170 minus your age). After five minutes, ride at your full speed for five to ten minutes. Your goal should be pedaling at sixty to eighty rpm's. Decrease your speed gradually to wind down your ride with a five-minute warm-down. This program should be repeated four times a week, increasing your time spent at full speed gradually. As your conditioning improves, you will find you have to increase the intensity of your exercise to maintain your training pulse rate.

Since most cities are poorly adapted to the use of bicycles, extra precautions should be taken to avoid accidents. As with most activities, having the proper conditioning and appropriate equipment will reduce the likelihood of injuries occurring. For night riding, you should have reflectors and head-light attachments on your bicycle, in addition to wearing reflectorized pieces of clothing. Helmets should also be worn (statistics show head injuries account for most fatal cycling injuries). Bike paths should be used whenever possible. However, since bikers usually share the roadways with cars, trucks, and motorcycles, a cyclist must be alert while riding in traffic. An alert rider is also a courteous one. Most cycle-car accidents are caused by the carelessness of the biker. Ignored traffic regulations and thoughtlessness contribute to the number of accidents. Losing control accounts for most biking accidents, from hitting holes and bumps to panic caused by being in traffic.

In the event of an accident while cycling, there are some guidelines for first aid that are helpful—immobilization, compression, and elevation (ICE). Immobilization reduces the risk of additional injuries, while compression with an elastic bandage can reduce swelling and bleeding. Be careful not to tie the bandage too tightly, or you may obstruct the blood flow. Elevation limits the initial injury and helps to decrease the swelling. Applying an ice pack or cold compress also provides pain relief and reduces swelling.

Racquetball

Fast becoming a national pastime, racquetball also offers terrific aerobic conditioning. In racquetball, you utilize short bursts of activity followed by brief periods of inactivity. Maintaining a high level of aerobic fitness is essential for the endurance involved in the game. Racquetball is the youngest of the racquet sports and can be enjoyed thoroughly at any level of competition. Besides being fun, racquetball is ideal for helping people achieve an aerobic fitness and for already athletic people who would like to stay in condition. It is a competitive game in which racquets are used to serve and return the ball. It may be played by two, three, or four players. To serve the ball, a player bounces it on the floor and strikes it so that it hits against the front wall and rebounds in back of the short line on the court. The objective is to serve or return the ball in such a way that your opponent cannot return the ball without bouncing it twice on the floor. A racquetball court has four walls. It is twenty feet wide, twenty feet high, and forty feet long. It is divided into a front and back court, which is separated by the short line, which should evenly divide the floor of the court. The grips involved in playing racquetball are the forehand and the backhand. You should grip the handle of your racquet so that the "V" formed by the thumb and forefinger is directly on top of the handle. A game is won with the scoring of twenty-one points.

Besides having a racquet, ball, and partner(s), you should also buy some additional equipment for playing racquetball. Buy a good pair of gym shoes that have a nonslip sole. Socks should be worn to avoid blistering. Shorts and T-shirts can be worn for clothing. As with tennis, the clothing should allow freedom of movement without being too baggy. Headbands and wristbands help cut down perspiration to eyes and hands. Eye injury is a real possibility, since the ball travels at high speeds and the playing space is confined. Eyeguards or goggles can be worn to cut down the possibility of getting injured in the eyes. The racquets are metal framed, and going to a pro shop will help you in your choice by consulting the sales personnel.

Like other sports, the proper conditioning and alertness will contribute to avoiding the likelihood of an accident. Keep out of your partner's way and know where the ball is at all times. Since most racquet sports are played in a half-crouch position, with the knees half-flexed and the lower back extended, there is a definite strain placed on the back and knees. Knee bends and torso stretches can help limber up your muscles before a game.

There are over 2,000 racquetball clubs with over 14 million players nationwide. Choosing your club can be determined by various means. Talking to members of the club and the staff can help you find out what the facilities are and the cost. Most memberships range in price from $60 to $350 per year. This may include additional features such as indoor tracks, weight rooms and heated pools. You may check into seeing whether a separate price is available for racquetball privileges only.

Injuries similar to tennis can occur while playing racquetball. Achilles tendonitis comes from overuse of an unconditioned muscle and can be relieved by resting the affected area. Sprains, pulls, and inflammations all arise from an overstress or improper technique. Again, it is important to have the proper warm-up and warm-down exercises such as jumping jacks, toe touches, and side stretches to increase your flexibility.

Tennis

One of the most enjoyable exercises with aerobic benefits is tennis. You can determine the level of competition you would like to play at or simply play for your own enjoyment. The muscles strengthened by a game of tennis are your shoulders, forearms (playing arm only), thighs, and calf muscles. Being very dynamic in movements, the benefits aerobically are many. The cardiovascular system is placed under great stress to meet the extra muscle demands during a game of tennis. Since tennis does expend a lot of energy, I do not recommend it to those of you who have remained sedentary for many years. Physical fitness allows for a better game and aerobic benefits. An unconditioned player will fatigue easy, putting unnecessary strain on his heart. The calorie usage in tennis can be a very effective weight control. A game of doubles uses up about 300 calories per hour, while playing singles will burn off 450 calories per hour.

For those of you who wish to resume playing tennis, or are conditioned enough to start, there are some helpful hints that can be of aid. First, reevaluate your playing style to accommodate physical changes. You do not have the body of a twenty-year old anymore, but the senior competitor can compensate with his experience, skill, mental attitude, and ball placement. Establish realistic goals for yourself. Know your limitations both physically and mentally, and work on your strong points.

Your body needs time to condition, and tennis involves more than physical fitness. Many skills go into a successful game. Accuracy is a major factor. The accurate placement of the ball as well as anticipating your opponent's ball placement is very important. Accuracy in placing the ball can be improved by playing alone against a backboard. Another exercise to help you practice on ball placement is to place an object in the far court and try to hit it while serving. This target practice not only helps your accuracy, but your serving ability as well. Putting the ball where you want it to go can be worked on through practice. With concentration and determination, all tennis skills can be improved.

Joining a club is another way of improving your game. Most clubs run from $150 to at least $200 per year in membership fees. Investigate the club first, comparing prices, asking someone who is already a member his opinion of the club, and find out how much individual instruction is offered or how large classes are for group instruction. Depending on the individual club, additional fees may be charged for court time and lessons. In choosing a teacher, make sure you feel comfortable around him. You will be spending a lot of time with each other and should check to see if his personality and teaching style are compatible with you. A teacher should help you learn (or relearn) the basics of tennis, as well as improving your skills.

Tennis gear should be bought at a pro shop. They usually offer the best merchandise at the most value and have a knowledgeable staff to assist you in your choice of equipment. Rackets come in wood, metal, fiberglass, and composite materials. Choose a racket suitable to your style and technique. A wood racket allows for a lot of control in hitting the ball, but little power. Although wood rackets are usually lower in price, they tend to wear down with use. Metal rackets give you a lot of power but little control. Fiberglass and composite rackets (made of wood and fiberglass) offer the best qualities of power and control. They are also hard to break, resist impact stress well and are inexpensive. Most rackets are subject to warping, so you need to purchase a press or square framework to lock over the face when the racket is not in use. Choose a racket that is not too heavy and will weigh you down as you play. Also make sure the grip is good. Stringing the racket again should be suited to your individual needs. A hard hitter needs a stiff frame with high-tension stringing. A racket can be strung to your needs, with light to heavy tension. The average player should have his racket strung at fifty-four to fifty-six pounds per square inch of tension. Strings can be made of a natural catgut material or of a nylon, manmade fiber. Natural strings come in a variety of thickness, types, and prices. They are very durable but easily affected by the weather. They tend to absorb moisture, deadening the tightness. Manmade strings do not absorb moisture, wear well, and can be made stretchproof.

Balls are uniformly pressure balls and tend to leak pressure once hit by the racket or the ground. Old balls are good for practicing with, though bad habits and technique may develop from overplaying a dead ball. There are many courts available to play on. A grass court gives very fast play, as the ball does not grip the surface. On a clay court, the ball does grip the surface, allowing for a much slower play. On concrete courts you lose the slowness of a clay court and gain speed, though the pounding of your feet on the hard surface makes one prone to injuries. A synthetic surface such as astroturf is faster than clay but not as fast as a grass court.

The shoes you wear should be chosen accordingly to the type of court you will most likely be playing on. You need a good gripping sole for playing on a grass or clay court, since you tend to slide easily. For concrete and synthetic courts, you need a rugged face sole and one that gives good support. Fabric and mesh material shoes are not as durable as leather shoes, but lighter in weight. Again, going to a tennis pro shop will help you in your selection.

Clothing should allow freedom of movement and be lightweight. Light cotton wear is best. Socks help reduce chafing and headbands and wristbands help in absorbing perspiration. In choosing the clothes for your game, do not sacrifice comfort for design. The old rule of white only still applies in some clubs; you'd better check first.

Flexibility, proper warm-up and warm-down exercises, conditioning, and proper technique all help to prevent injuries. Tennis requires flexibility in the torso and upper body. The knees and arms are also used extensively. Stretching exercises such as sit-ups, knee bends, toe touching, arm extensions, neck twists, and leg stretches all help in increasing a player's flexibility. Dumbbell curls (pronating and supinating) with the arms and leg raises help to strengthen the muscles used in a game of tennis. Strengthening the abdomen, buttocks, and thigh muscles helps take the strain off the back. Short-distance running and agility drills, such as running sideways from one side of the court to the other, are good training exercises. Slow stretching parts of the body gradually lengthens the ligaments and muscle/tendon units.

The injuries one can incur while playing tennis can also be worked on. Properly warming-up and flexibility exercising and lightweight training exercises should help to relieve shoulder injuries. Overstretching and overworking the muscles and tendons in the arm and elbow results in *tennis elbow*. This is tendonitis of the muscles on the back of the arm at the elbow. This can be prevented by proper weight training and a correction in technique. *Tennis knee* is an irritation of the cartilage of the knee joint that deep-knee bends can help you avoid. *Tennis leg* is a tear of the calf muscle on the inner side of the leg. This usually happens from turning to strike a sudden backhand. Resting the leg until you can walk with no pain is the best treatment.

In addition to all the activities mentioned, there are many others that can give beneficial aerobic conditioning. Mountain climbing, hiking, brisk walking, rowing and paddling, and conditioning calisthenics are all good exercises that increase your aerobic conditioning and endurance. Common sense should be used in whichever activity you choose. Overtaxing and straining yourself will only lead to fatigue and defeat the purpose of an aerobic program. Straining yourself without the proper conditioning in any sport or activity can also do more damage than good. Remember that most injuries and accidents can be avoided with the proper equipment, warming-up and warming-down exercises, and strengthening exercises particular to the activity. I recommend swimming and bicycling for those who are prohibited from running or a more strenuous sport due to health or heart problems. A general rule you can use in any aerobic exercise is to remember that the intensity must be increased gradually for you to benefit from aerobic endurance.

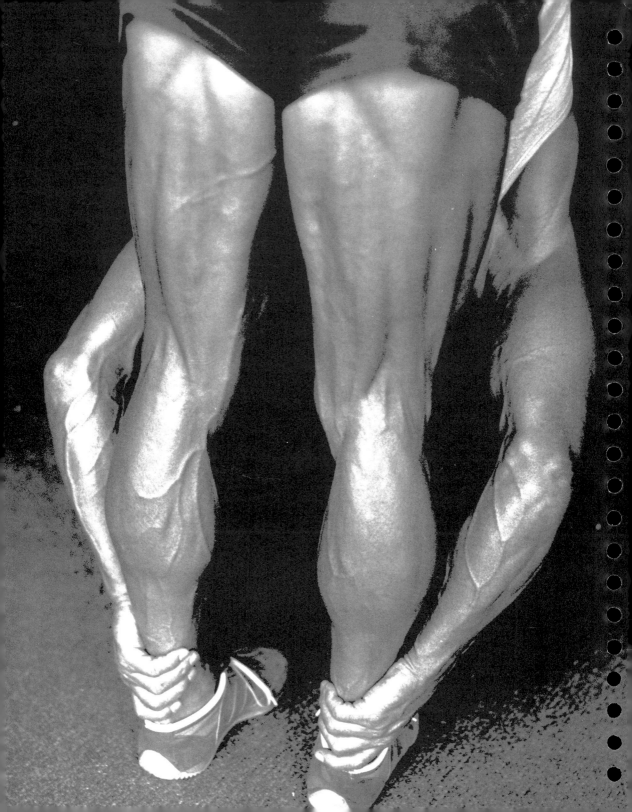

FLEXIBILITY

Stretching has fortunately become more popular the last few years, partially due to the media focusing in on different aspects of sports, including all the different training regimens. There are numerous books and articles on stretching. This chapter will give you the basic stretching exercises for increasing your flexibility, but it is not a complete listing of all the stretches there are. I feel what you are given here is adequate, but if you want to research stretching exercises more, you will find that there are literally hundreds of stretches.

If you are performing any weight-training routines, this chapter on flexibility is important to you, so don't just skip over it! To get the most out of your weight training, as well as your aerobic activities, you need to stretch for three to six minutes both before and after your workout, game, or run. Your stretching regimen should be part of your warming up as well as cooling down. Stretching is especially crucial before your leg routine and before running. If you are not stretched out, you might strain a muscle or get what is commonly called a hamstring pull.

Stretching out will help to prevent injuries and will also help you from becoming stiff and immobile. Especially now that you are getting older, stretching will help you from becoming stiff and bent up. When you get older, you tend to lose the mobility you had when you were younger. And it's not just losing a step; your body is almost freezing up. But this doesn't have to happen if you follow a good stretching routine. Just pick from one to two exercises per body part to do each day. You don't have to limit yourself to stretching only when you are working out or when you are going to run or play a game. You can do it in your home every day. Just be sure to start slowly, don't jerk, and don't hold the stretched position for more than a few seconds.

When you lift weights, you are contracting your muscles. When you stretch out, you are performing the needed opposite of the contracting movement. This principle is similar to positive and negative movements in your lifting. Stretching will not only increase your flexibility but it will make you feel better, so pick out your exercises, the ones you know you need, and get started right away! If you have time to lift weights or play sports, you have time to stretch.

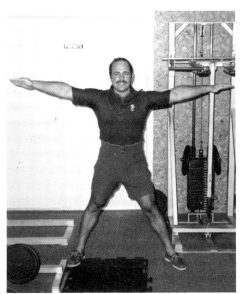

A1: Circular Shoulder Rotation
Rotate the neck in a full circle, extending the head as far back as it will go. Use the same motion for the arms and trunk, completing at least 10 full circles. These exercises will loosen up the key muscle groups.

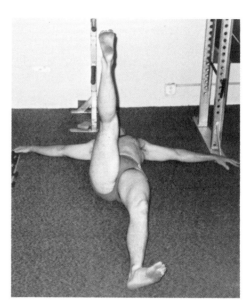

B1-2: Hamstring Trunk Rotation
This should be done with both legs straight and your hands on the ground. Attempt to touch your right foot to the left hand and the left foot to the right hand. Stretch the hamstrings 2 to 3 times in this manner.

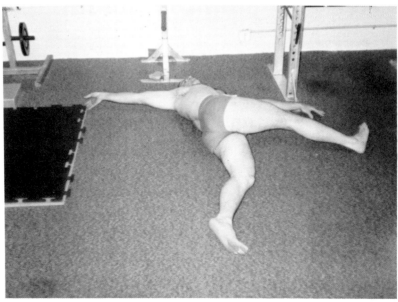

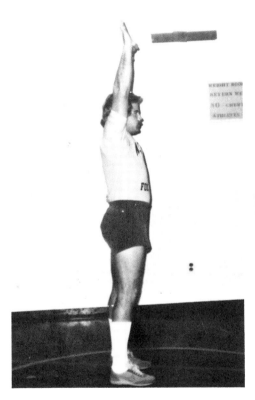

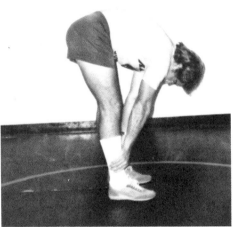

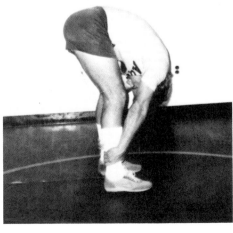

C1-3: Hamstring Stretch I (left)
This exercise will loosen up the hamstring muscle, which together with the quadricep provides 80 percent of the knee's support. With hands fully extended into the air, bend over, being careful not to bend your knees. The motion should be a smooth movement. Be careful not to jerk down and pull the hamstrings. Grasp your ankles and continue the motion until your head touches your knees.

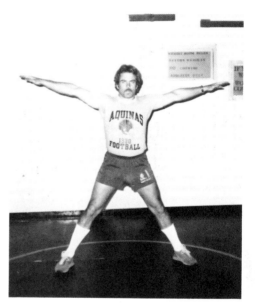

D1-2: Hamstring Stretch II
Start in a position such as the one used in the circular shoulder rotation but this time spread the legs as far apart as possible. Grasp the ankle with both hands and attempt to touch your chin to your knee. Repeat with both legs 2 to 3 times.

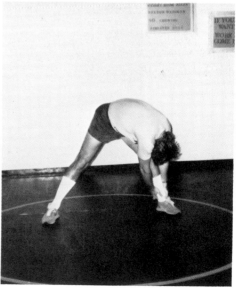

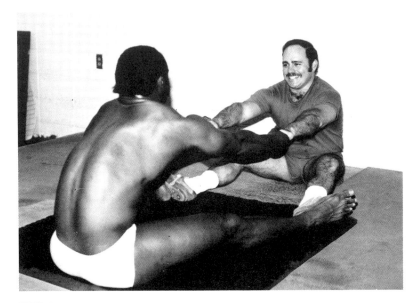

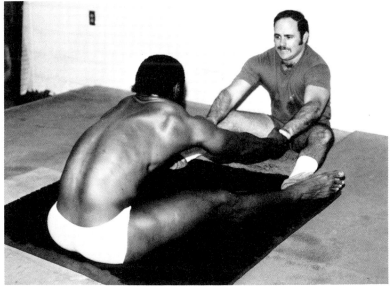

E1-2: Partner Stretch
With your partner facing you, stretch open the legs until your feet touch the inside of his ankles. While grasping each other's wrists, pull back while your partner offers resistance. Repeat the exercise with reversed roles.

F1: Flip-Over Hamstring Stretch
Lying flat on the ground with your hands at your side, lock the knees and spread your legs as far apart as possible. Raise your legs until your toes touch the ground. Those suffering from lower-back problems should avoid this exercise.

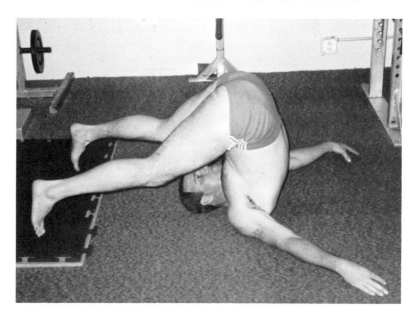

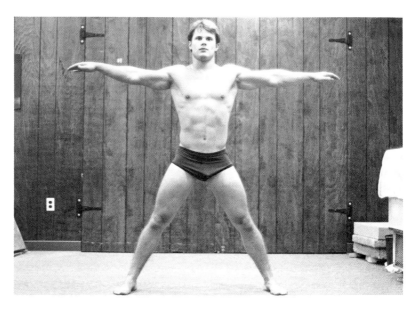

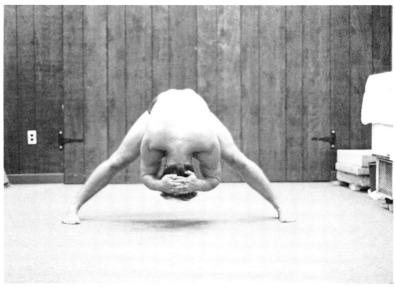

G1-2: Bent-Over Hamstring Stretch

Starting in the spread-eagle position, place your hands behind your head and attempt to touch the ground with your head. Stretch slowly and avoid jerking.

H1: Hamstring Groin Stretch I

Place your leg at a right-angle position and grasp the ankle of the horizontal leg while attempting to touch your chin to your knee.

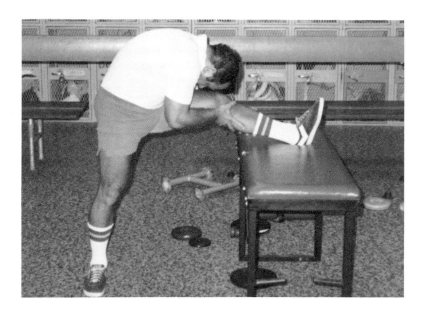

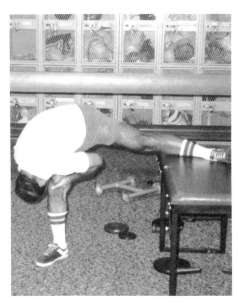

I1: Hamstring Groin Stretch II
Starting in the same position as the previous exercise, grasp the ankle of the standing leg and touch the chin to your knee while keeping your knees straight.

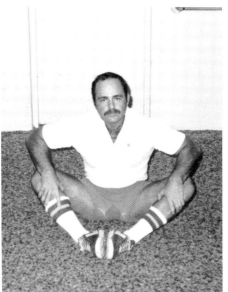

J1: Lotus Groin Stretch
Position yourself with ankles meeting and hands on your knees. Push down on the knees and try to touch them to the ground.

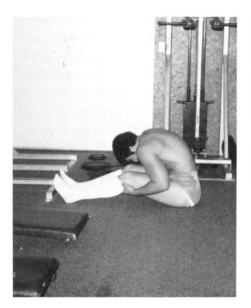

K1: Hamstring Lower-Back Stretch *(left, top)*
Beginning in a sitting position, grasp behind the calf and try to touch your forehead to your knees. Be carefeul not to bounce down; rather, do it in one easy motion to maximize the benefit to the hamstring and lower back.

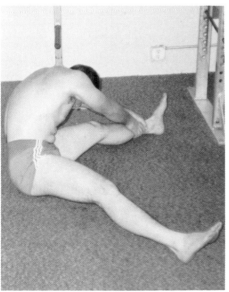

L1: Modified Hurdler's Stretch
With both legs spread apart, keep the knee touching the ground and then attempt to touch your forehead to your knee.

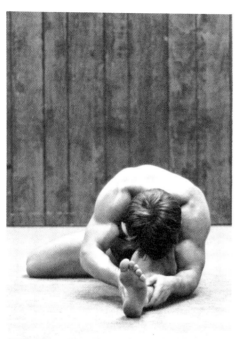

M1: Hurdler's Stretch
Change your position slightly
from the previous exercise by
bending one knee while keeping
the legs apart at a right angle.
Stretch the hamstrings by
leaning forward on your straight
leg while you try to keep the
knee touching the ground to
stretch the quadriceps.

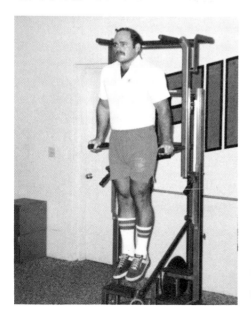

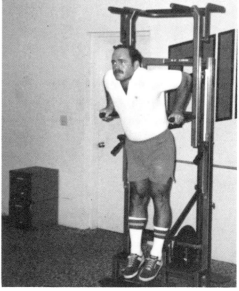

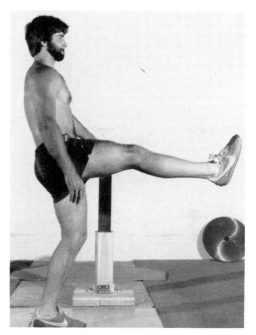

N1-2: Negative Dip *(below left)*
This is the finest stretching
exercise for upper-body
flexibility. Just raise yourself up
on the dipping bar and then let
yourself down slowly, doing the
negative aspect of the dip only.

O1-2: Leg Extension
Extend your leg in all possible
positions, keeping the knee stiff.
You may need some help from a
partner to get the full extension.

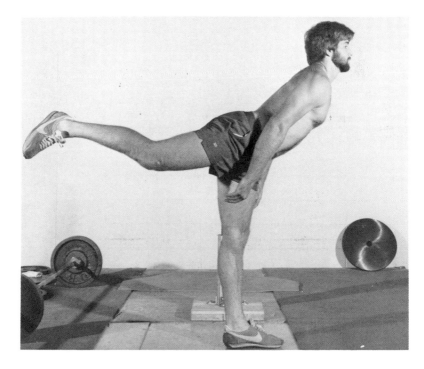

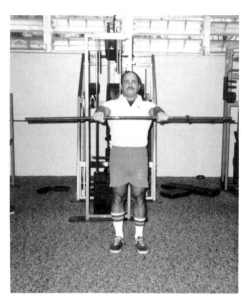 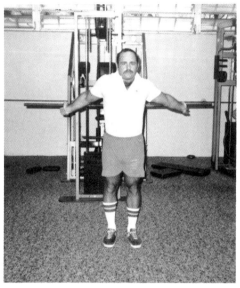

P1-2: Bar Stretch
Hold a bar at the ends in front
of you at shoulder height.
Extend the bar slowly over your
head and down to waist level.

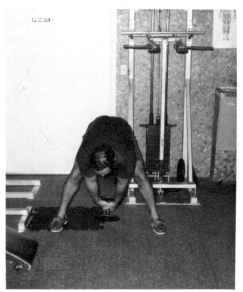 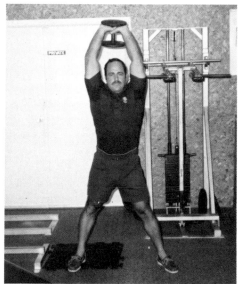

Q1-2: Dumbbell Swing
This is actually a great warm-up exercise that affects about every muscle group in the body. Start with a very light weight. Stand comfortable with your feet about 1½-2 feet apart. Hold the dumbbell with a hand-over-hand safe grip and, in a crouched squat, start with the dumbbell down between your legs. With a swift swing, move the dumbbell out in front of you to either chin high or, if the weight is very light, over your head in a standing position. Then let the dumbbell swing down while you crouch back to the starting position. Exhale as you swing up and inhale as you go down. Do sets of 12 to 20.

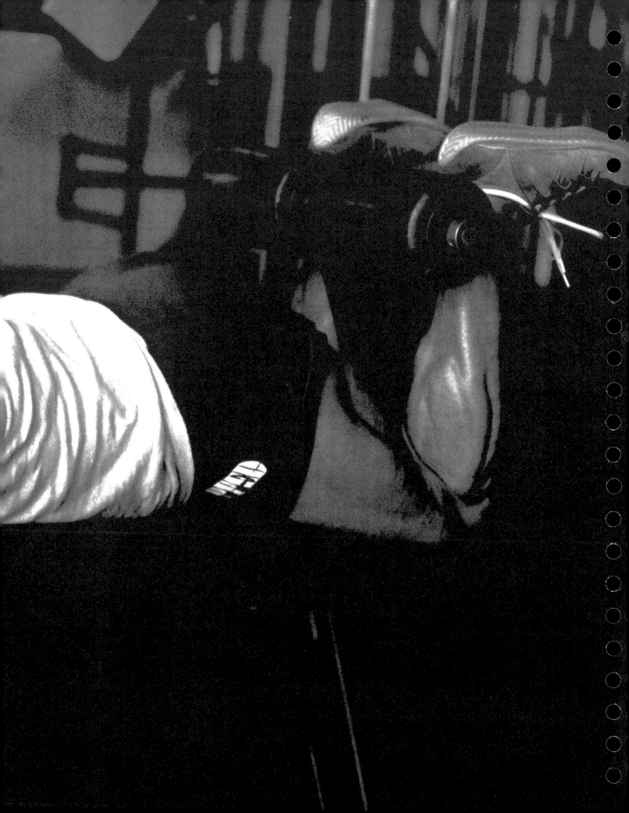

LEGS

You can't support a big body on little pins! It is depressing to me, as a coach, to see so many weight trainers concentrating on building up the upper body and neglecting the legs. When I asked them why they were not working their legs, they said that they were running for their legs. Running is not enough for your legs! Running is great for cardiovascular conditioning, general body tone, and absolutely necessary for athletes, but it is not enough. You might notice that Olympic sprinters have outstanding legs, but they have a grueling sprint workout that quickly contracts the muscle and builds them up. I don't think many of you would like to have legs that look like a long-distance runner's legs. They have very thin legs without much muscular definition. That is because their unbelievable workouts of running long distances breaks down their leg muscles and doesn't allow them to build up size. Those long distances burn up lots of calories and keep them thin. Probably most of them are ectomorphs, (thin type build with small- or medium-sized bones) anyway and would find it harder than most to build up size. I don't mean to give long-distance runners a bad rep because they probably have the hardest training routine of any athlete. It is just that their legs are generally not aesthetic or what you would want to strive for.

The major muscles in the legs are the gluteus maximus (hips); the posterior thigh muscles, the majority of which are the hamstrings (hams), which are also called thigh biceps; anterior thigh muscles, which grouped together are generally called the quadriceps even though they also include the vastus group, etc.; and the calf, which includes the gastrocnemius (major part of the calf and should be diamond shaped) and the soleus, which is the lower part of the calf.

Older men's legs seem to lose their shape rather quickly after they get out of school. An important reason for the man over thirty-five to perform leg work is that it speeds up your metabolism, burns up a lot of calories in high repetitions, and helps your whole body's strength to increase. Performing leg work will help to counteract, to some extent, the slowing down of your metabolism when you get older. If you just performed leg work alone, it would help to shape up your whole body and tone you up.

Tom Platz, one of the world's top bodybuilders, has the most amazing set of legs in the world. He has repeatedly stated that the key to his fantastic legs is squats. Squat, squat, squat!!! The squat is a basic, but tremendous, exercise. It is the most beneficial exercise for your body in all of weight training. It not only works the glutes, quads, and hams, but it helps to expand your rib cage and gets the blood flowing. Squatting will help your total strength and, amazingly enough, will help your maximum lift in the bench press to go up. It works the legs and back in unison, as you do in sports. High-repetition squats are good for cardiovascular conditioning and will burn up lots of calories. You will find that it is the most taxing of all exercises, and you will have to go slower than in the other exercises.

Squats have a bad reputation in some circles—some saying that they are dangerous to your back and knees. If they were so dangerous, why do most professional football teams have their players do them? Surely they wouldn't risk damaging their great investments by having them do something that might be harmful to them. As long as you are warmed up first and go down slowly, keeping your back straight, you won't hurt your back. You might hurt your back if you descended quickly or bent over too much. If you are warmed up and don't go below the point in which your thighs are parallel to the floor and don't bounce, you shouldn't hurt your knees. It's when you bounce up that you could hurt your knees. Another criticism of squats is that they reportedly build up your butt too much. Squats do work your glutes (butt) but will tighten them and give them a good shape along with working the rest of your legs. If you have found in middle age that your hind end is bigger with more fat than when you were younger, squats would be great to firm up those glutes. Squats will not give you a fat butt. Vince Gironda, a bodybuilding guru with his own ideas, believes in doing hack squats instead of regular squats in order to avoid working the glutes. A hack squat is a fine exercise, especially for the quads, but can't compare with the regular squat. If you followed the theory that you should avoid squats in order not to develop a big butt, then you should avoid sit-ups and leg raises in order not to get a big stomach.

If you have knee problems, you should consult with a sports physician about squatting, just as you would if you had another body part injured. In most cases, after considerable therapy, you can return to at least partial if not parallel squats. I suffered a torn anterior cruciate ligament recently playing handball, but after quality therapy by Steve Antonopolus at the Denver Bronco headquarters, I returned to partial squats after six weeks and parallel squats after three months.

Leg extensions really bring those quads out. If you don't have a quad machine, you can use iron boots. Leg curls will bomb those hams. Your hams should be two-thirds as strong as your quads, so if you are using 100 pounds on your leg extensions, you should be using between 65 and 70 pounds on your leg curls. A leg press is a good compound leg exercise—that is, it works both the anterior and posterior thigh muscles together. But be careful because it can put more strain on your knees than a squat, depending on how you use it. An old-fashioned exercise that I have also been using of late is the lunge. If you think your hams and lower glute tie-ins have been worked before, just try this exercise and I promise you that you will be sore. But avoid this if you have any knee problems.

If I have seen 1,000 neglected thighs, I have seen 2,000 neglected calves. The calves are one of the muscle groups that seem to atrophy first in the older man. The reason for that is because of the decrease in the running, walking, stair climbing, and sports when you get older. The calves are the hardest muscle group in your body to build up, mainly because you are already using them constantly in walking, climbing stairs, and getting up from a seated position. Because they are so hard to build up, you really have to work through the pain. I recommend doing ten burning reps (you only start counting when you start to burn). Because you are using these muscles constantly, like abdominals, they are one of the very few muscle groups you can work every day. Some people believe in high reps and others in a few heavy reps. Whatever works for you is fine, but I recommend getting to those burns quickly, which would necessitate using a heavy weight. I like donkey toe raises the best because the weight is so close to your calves and mostly because they seem to pump the gastrocnemius the best. To hit the lower part of the calf (soleus), I use a seated calf machine.

If you do a three-day leg workout, make sure that you have only one heavy day, one medium day, and one light day. Otherwise you will be overtrained. Believe it or not, it's just as easy to overtrain as undertrain.

Because tennis, racquetball, and running are great strains on your legs, performing leg work with weights will help to prevent knee and other leg injuries. Eighty percent of the support for your knee comes the quadriceps and hamstrings. When you build those up, you reduce the chance of a serious knee injury. An ounce of prevention is worth a pound of cure. You are born with so much speed; you have or you don't. However, you can improve your speed a little by building your leg strength through weight training. Increased speed will certainly help your tennis and racquetball as well as give you an added help for your races, if you are in any. Leg work will also help your bicycling and endurance for biking. Your swimming will also be improved because your leg strength is an important part of swimming.

The reason I have legs at the beginning of the body parts is two fold. One is because I believe it is the most important and overlooked muscle group. The other reason is because I believe you should start your workouts with your largest muscle groups first. Your legs are the largest muscle groups in your body, and leg work is the most taxing, so get it done first or you might not have the strength to do it at the end of your workout. By working the largest muscle groups first, you are following a logical and kinesiologically correct procedure.

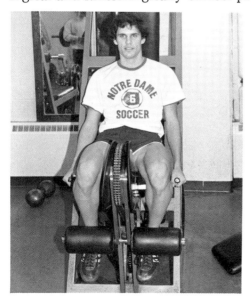 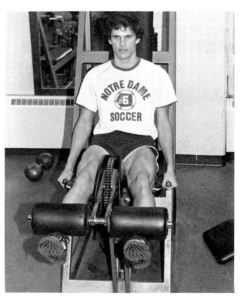

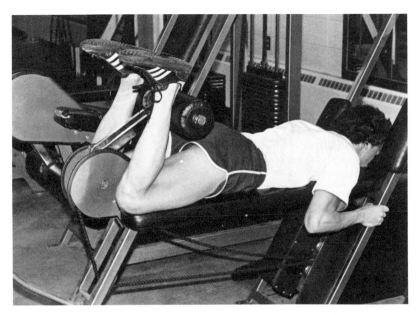

A1-2: Nautilus Leg Extension
(left)
In a seated position, place your feet behind the roller pads with your knees snug against the seat. Make sure to keep your head and shoulders against the seat back. Straighten both of your legs smoothly. Pause. Slowly lower your resistance and repeat. It is important that you avoid tightly gripping the handles and gritting the teeth, tensing the neck and face muscles when you move.

B1: Nautilus Leg Curl
Lie face down on the machine and place your feet under the roller pads with your knees just over the edge of the bench. Lightly grasp the handles to keep your body from moving and then curl your legs, trying to touch your heels to your buttocks. When your lower legs are perpendicular to the bench, lift your buttocks to increase your movement. Then pause at the point of full muscular contraction. Slowly lower your resistance and repeat the exercise.

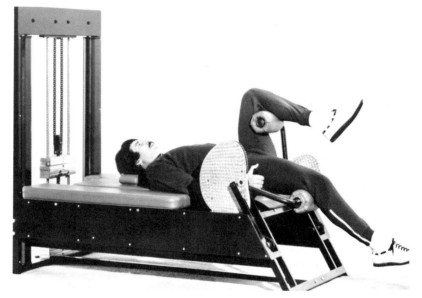

**C1: Nautilus Hip-and-Back
Machine**
Lie on your back, shoulders
against the pads. Strap the seat
belt around your waist and
grasp the handles while placing
your legs over the pads so that
the knees are close to the chest.
Straighten your legs out while
keeping the back straight.

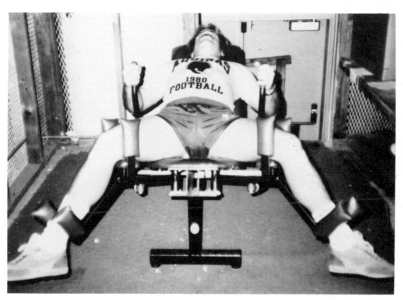

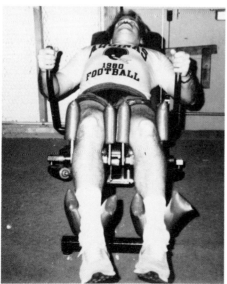

D1-2: Hydra-Gym Ad-Ab Machine

This is great for the inner and outer parts of your thighs. In the starting position with your legs together, bring them out as fast and as hard as you can, then bring them together and repeat. Start with 2 sets of 20-seconds with a minute to rest. Then after you are broken in (after a couple of weeks), try 2 sets of 30-seconds.

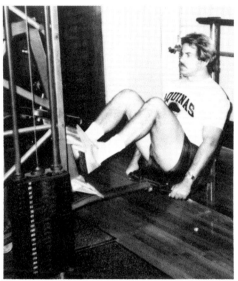 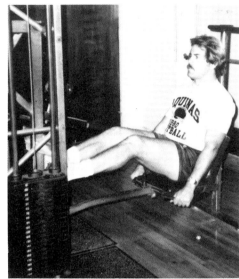

E1-2: Universal Leg Press
Adjust the support chair until
your legs bend as indicated.
Take a deep breath and push
with your legs until almost fully
extended but not locked out,
exhaling as you exert. Return to
the starting position and repeat.
If you are recuperating from
knee problems, be careful—
consult your physician before
doing the leg press.

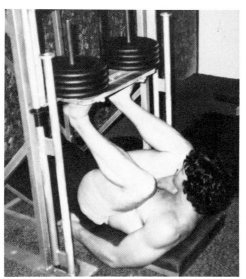 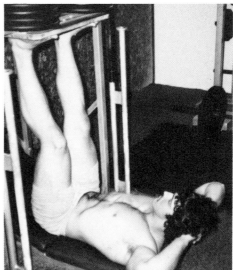

F1-2: Old-Fashioned Leg Press
Not recommended for anyone
recuperating from a knee injury.
Once again, fully extend the leg
12 times a set, completing 3 sets.
This machine puts pressure on
the knee, but it can be used in
conjunction with other leg
exercises.

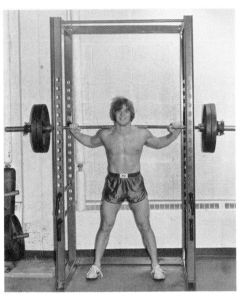 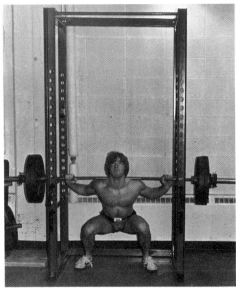

G1-2: Squat

Place the weight behind the neck. This squat works the posterior and anterior thigh muscles, the gluteus maximus, and even the rib cage. Lower yourself slowly to avoid back injury, and don't bounce off the knee. Be careful if you have knee problems; consult your physician first. You may have to do partial squats instead of complete ones (where the thighs are parallel to the ground) if you have knee problems.

H1-2: Front Squat *(right)*

Front squats will help you strengthen your quadriceps. Start by resting the weight on your shoulders in an upright position, arms crossed to hold the barbell. Lower yourself until your thighs are parallel to the floor. Remember to keep your back straight and your head up while you lower yourself. Don't bounce into the lower position. The success of this exercise relies on lowering yourself slowly.

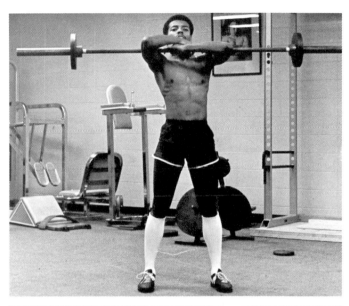

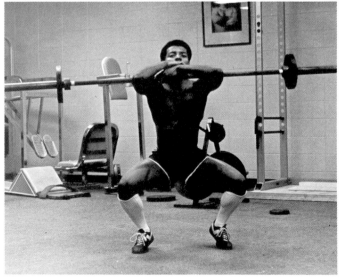

I1-2: Hack Squat

Grip the bar behind your back
in a downward position and
then raise up to a three-quarters
position. Then move down until
your thighs are parallel to the
ground. Make sure you come up
only three-quarters of the way.
This exercise pumps the
quadriceps (anterior thigh
muscles) as well as some
posterior thigh muscles
effectively. Some bodybuilders
prefer this exercise to the regular
squat because it does not work
your glutes.

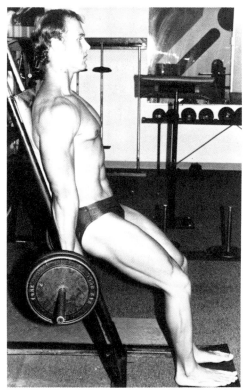

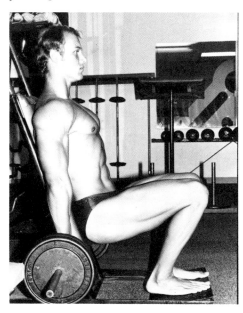

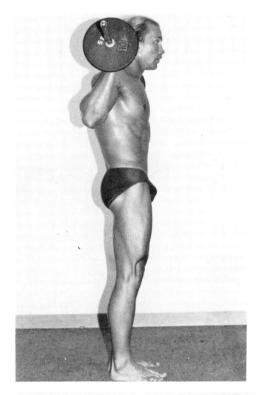

J1-2: Bar Lunge

Stand straight up with the bar resting on your back. Extend one leg forward and bend down until the opposite leg is almost touching the ground. Then stand up straight and lunge forward with the other leg. This exercise effectively pumps your thighs, especially the glute-ham tie-in.

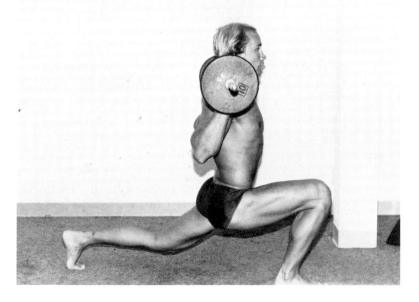

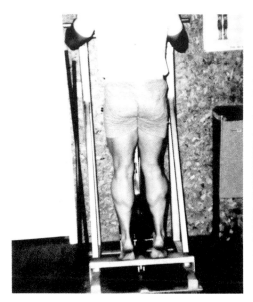

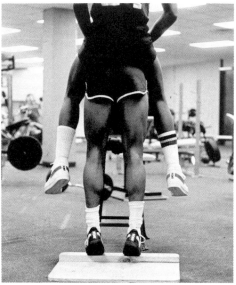

K1: Toe Raise
The calves are the target of this exercise, performed using this old-fashioned toe-raise machine. The development of the calves can increase a player's speed and quickness, and toe raises work on the calves with quick results. Try for a full extension as you thrust upward onto your toes.

L1: Donkey Toe Raise
Donkey toe raises are more difficult than regular toe raises because of the weight's closer proximity to the calves. Have a partner sit on your back as you brace yourself over a table. Thrust upwards onto your toes a minimum of 20 repetitions a set. You should feel that good "burning sensation" in the calves at least 10 times to utilize this exercise effectively.

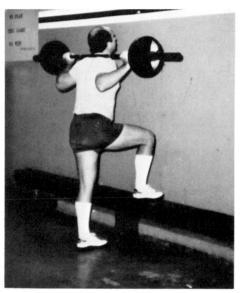 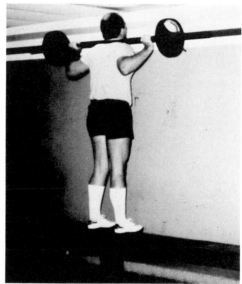

M1-2: Step Up

This is as easy as walking up
stairs. But avoid it if you have
leg or knee problems. With the
weight in the position as
indicated, just step up and down
a step. This is a good overall
thigh exercise. Don't use too
heavy a weight. Do in
repetitions of 12 to 15.

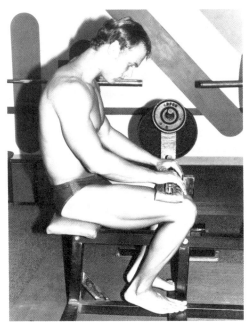 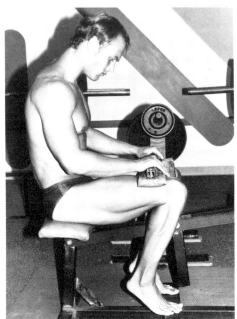

N1-2: Seated Calf-Toe Raise

Wedge your knees under the padded bar and move your heels up and down as far as possible. Fred Everts is shown doing this exercise on the seated calf machine. This exercise works your soleus, or the lower part of your calves. Make sure you do at least 10 burning reps.

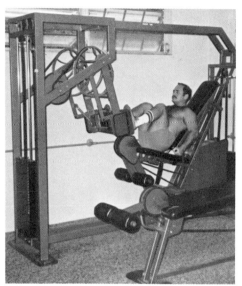 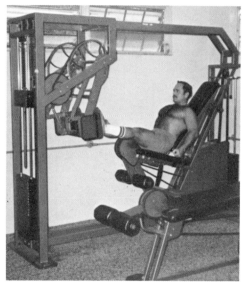

O1-2: Nautilus Compound Leg Machine
Seat yourself in the machine, knees bent and feet against the pads. Grasp the handles lightly. Press the legs forward to full extension, keeping the back against the seat.

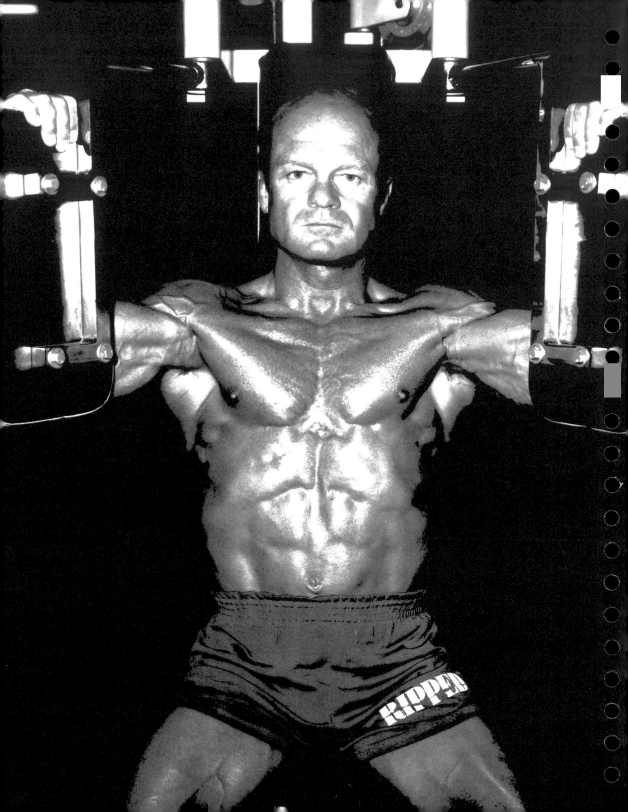

CHEST

Have you sadly noticed that your chest has seemed to sag since you have gotten older? Do your pectorals appear soft and seem to be hanging on your body? If the answer to these questions is yes, don't be too worried—it happens to most men as they get into middle age, and it's something that a good diet and the right weight-training exercises, such as plenty of dumbbell or cable flies, can rectify.

The chest is probably a close second to the arms in popularity for training. Manliness and big chests have long been equated. The largest part of the chest is the pectorals, major and minor. The rib cage and serratus magnus, a three-fingered muscle attached thereto, are also considered part of the chest. Many trainers feel that a rib cage (actually the cartilage) can't be expanded once a person is past the age of twenty-one, so they don't stress rib-cage expansion exercises like the pullover for older men. I believe that the rib cage can be expanded well past twenty-one, but I doubt whether you will be able to after thirty-five. However, since all heavy breathing exercises, such as squats, will expand the rib cage (which will give you the appearance of a barrel chest), if you are one of the few over thirty-five who can expand your rib cage, it will be developed by high repetition squats. Here we are on the chest, and I am still mentioning squats, but I told you they were the greatest exercise in weight training.

I have included bench presses in this section for simplicity. The bench press is an upper-body compound exercise that develops most of your upper body but primarily the deltoid, triceps, and the major part of your pectorals. However, I don't think it is the greatest exercise specifically for the chest. Between 30 and 38 percent of it works the pecs. The variation is due to where you hold your hands—the wider out, the more you work your pecs; the closer in, the more you work your triceps. The majority of the bench press works the deltoids and triceps. A side benefit of the close-grip bench press, which I have included under arms, is that it works the interior part of the pecs.

You could develop a massive chest with two exercises alone—the incline press (preferably with dumbbells) and the forward dip. The incline press works the upper pecs (besides deltoids and triceps), and the forward dip works the lower pecs as well as the outside of the pecs. The decline press is a supplementary exercise to develop the lower pecs. I recommend an angle of about 38 percent in the incline. Once you get 45 percent and more, you are getting too much deltoid development and too little in the upper pecs.

For mature men, I highly recommend flies. They square off your chest, and if you have the problem of a sagging chest that I described earlier, they will really help you. I would mix up all variety of flies—incline, flat, decline, cables, crossovers, etc. Of course you wouldn't do all types of flies at once, but through the routines you can mix them up in order to work all parts of your chest. For advanced trainees (and I mean advanced!), I like to superset my flies with inclines or declines. By exhausting the pecs first with the flies, then doing the compound exercise immediately after (no more than four seconds before each movement) like the inclines or declines, you get a real pump. The congestion from using this pre-exhaust principle is amazing. Advanced trainees can use this principle with almost any muscle groups by first doing the isolation exercise, then immediately doing the compound exercise.

Because of the popularity of chest work, you should be careful not to overtrain it. You want your body to look symmetrical. It would look absurd to have a great big and defined chest with the rest of your body small and underdeveloped.

Those of you who swim will find that not only your breast stroke improves when you develop your chest muscles but also your freestyle swimming. The pectorals are used in all your swimming motions. In racquetball and tennis, your backhand shots will be improved by developing your pecs.

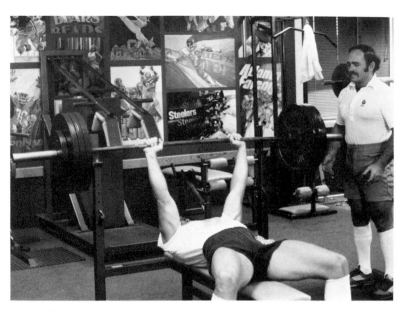

A1: Bench Press

Grasp the bar at shoulder width
and bring the bar down to the
top of your pectorals with an
inhaling breath; then press the
bar upwards as you exhale until
you can fully extend and lock
your arms. Do not arch your
back or buttocks but remain in
contact with the bench at all
times. Your feet should be flat
on the floor.

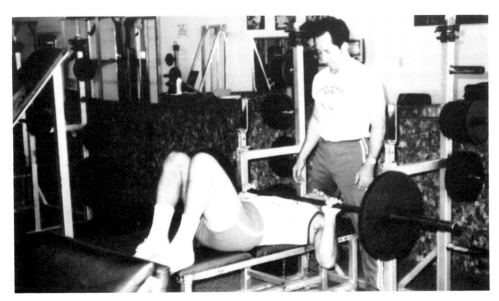

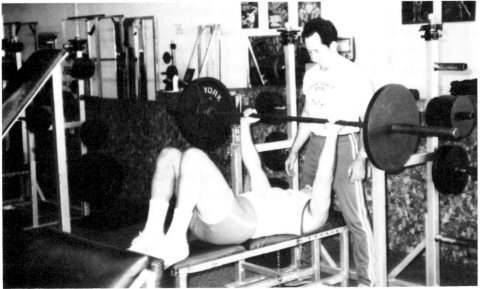

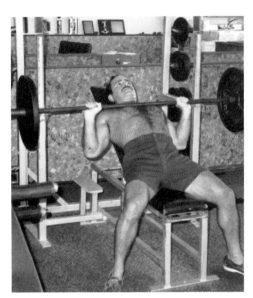 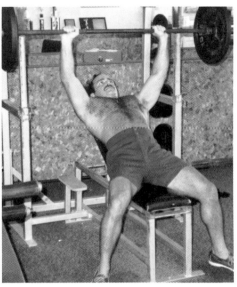

B1-2: Special Bench Press *(left)*
Bob Pure is shown doing the bench press this special way. By placing your feet up on the bench, you take away from any back strain. Otherwise the same instructions apply as to the regular bench press. Coach Rafael Guererro is shown spotting Bob.

C1-2: Barbell Incline Press
While at a 45° angle, press the bar upward with an exhaling breath, pausing to lock your arms in an extended position, and then lower the bar back down to the top of your pectorals. The incline press is also beneficial for building the pectoral-deltoid tie-in—an area of the upper chest that the bench press does not develop.

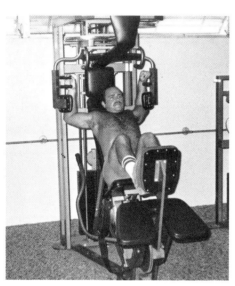
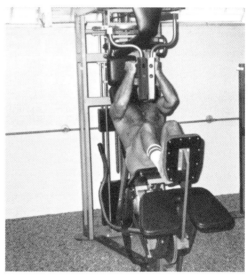
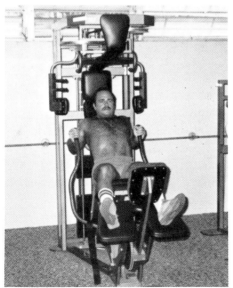
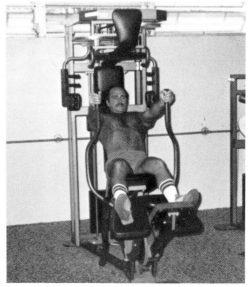

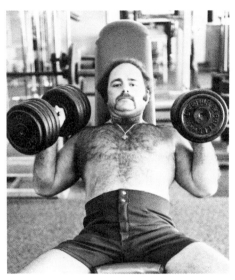 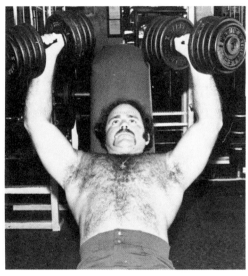

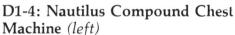

D1-4: Nautilus Compound Chest Machine *(left)*
Sit firmly in the chair and place your feet on the front pads. Put your forearms behind the pec-deck pads, grasping the handles. Smoothly bring the arms together, then apart. Now for the press portion of the exercise, rest your legs on the flat pads, grasping the press handles. Then press forward.

E1-2: Dumbbell Incline Press
This exercise strengthens the upper pectorals and triceps. It is especially effective for the pectoral-deltoid tie-in. Starting with the dumbbells wide apart yet touching your shoulders, press the dumbbells upwards until they are straight up and closer together than at the start.

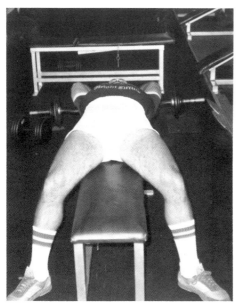 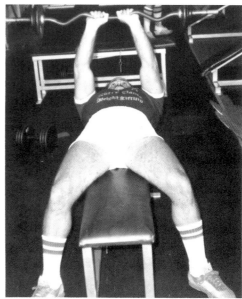

F1-4: Easy-Curl Pullover and Dumbbell Pullover

This strengthens the deltoids, lats, triceps, serratus magnus, and rib cage. It can be done using either an easy-curl bar or dumbbells. Lying either straight or across a bench with your head over the edge, pull the bar off the ground over your head to a position over the top of your pectorals. The hips must remain in contact with the bench throughout the exercise. It is also necessary to keep the bar or dumbbell from touching the pectorals, since this would reduce the muscle tension and take away from the effectiveness of the exercise. Avoid using a heavy weight for the pullover, for this will cause you to cheat by bending the elbows, which affects the lats more than the rib cage. Keep the rib cage relaxed, so you can stretch the entire rib structure.

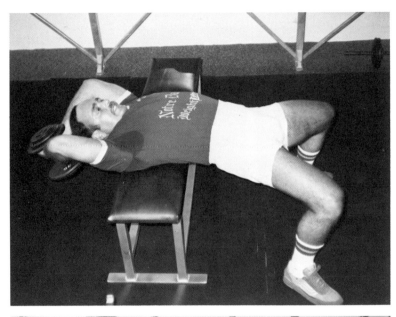

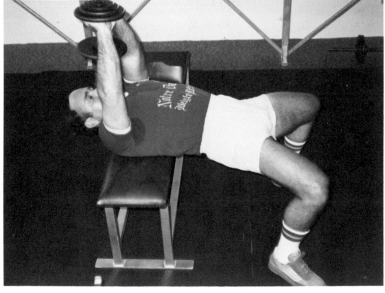

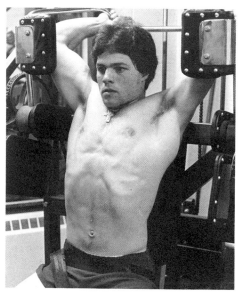 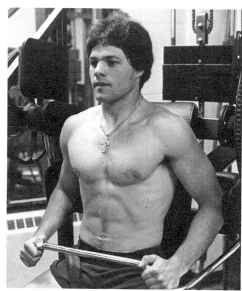

G1-2: Nautilus Pullover
Place the elbows on the pads
and rest your hands on the bar.
Pull the arms down to the fully
extended position.

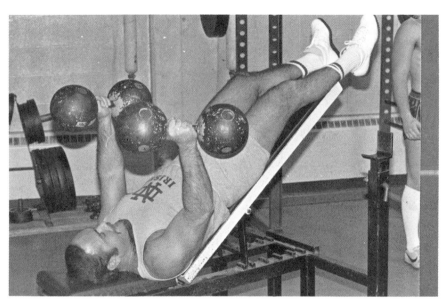

H1: Dumbbell Decline Press

This exercise works the lower
pectorals as well as the anterior
head of the deltoids and triceps.
Hold the dumbbells wide at the
base, touching your shoulders,
and press them up, narrow at
the top.

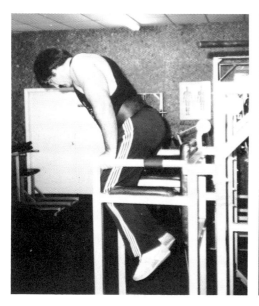

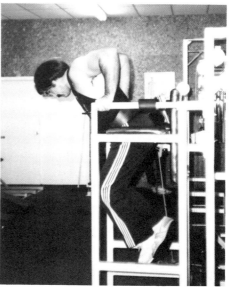

I1-2: Forward Dip
Lean forward and proceed to press yourself upwards while maintaining the forward lean. This will add bulk to the upper body and chest. You may use a dumbbell to weight yourself down.

J1-2: Flat Fly *(right)*
While lying flat on the bench with a dumbbell in each hand, extend your arms below the bench with your elbows slightly bent. Bring the two dumbbells up toward your chest (two-thirds of the way). You do not want to bring the dumbbells together because this would take the tension off. This exercise works to square off your middle pectorals (the major part of your chest) and the front and side heads of your deltoids.

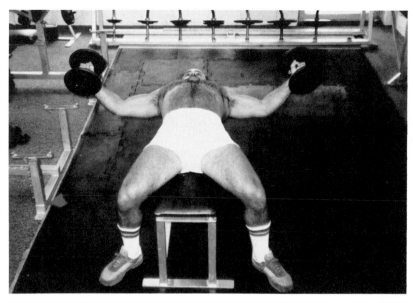

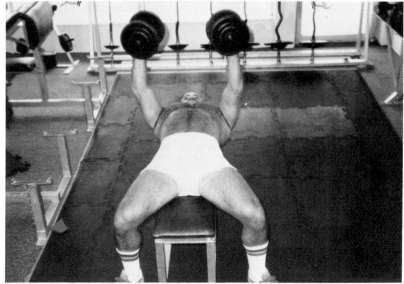

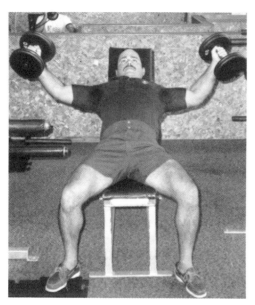 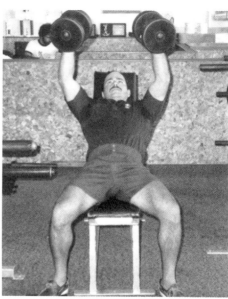

K1-2: Incline Fly
This exercise works the outer pectoral muscles. Keep your elbows bent slightly, and bring the dumbbells two-thirds to three-quarters of the way up across the chest. Don't lift the dumbbells all the way up until they touch, for that would release the tension on the outer pecs and minimize the efficiency of the exercise.

L1-2: Decline Fly *(right)*
At an angle of about 40°, extend your arms out as far as they can go, then bring them toward your chest middle until they are about three-quarters of the way together. Make sure you are secure in the decline bench. This really squares your lower and outer chest.

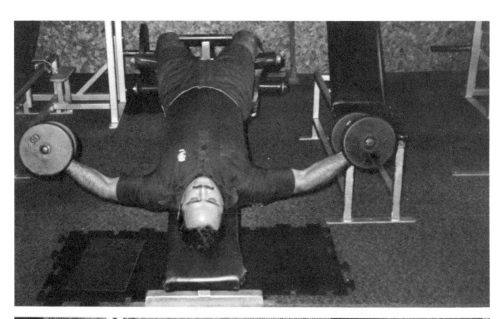

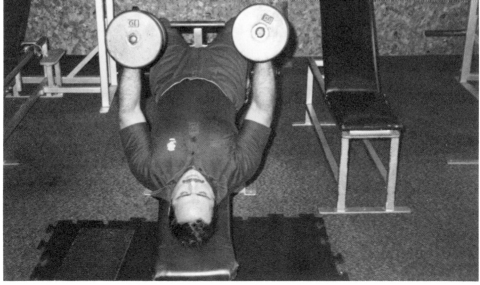

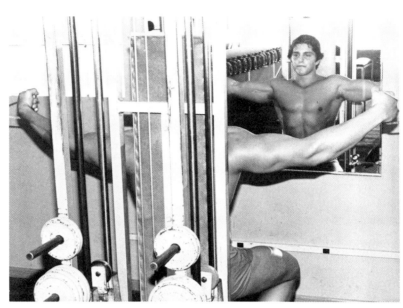

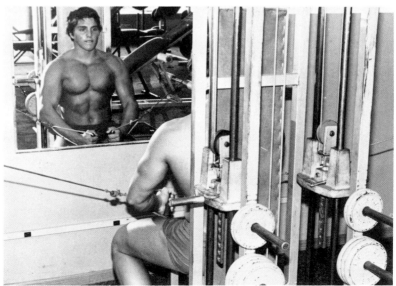

M1-3 Crossover Cable
In this exercise, you should be seated with your hands holding a cable. Extend your arms out fully to the side and bring the cables across your chest so that they cross each other. This is another advanced exercise that will square off your chest and pump your deltoids.

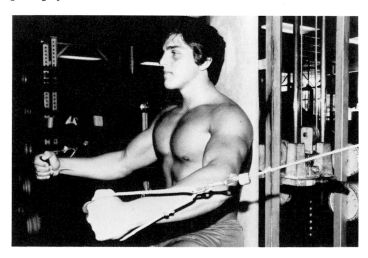

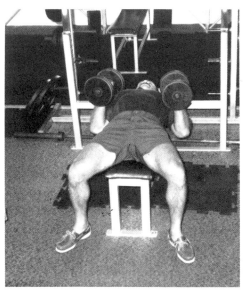 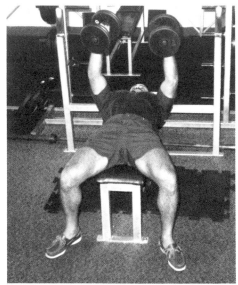

N1-2: Dumbbell Bench Press
Lie on a bench, holding
dumbbells shoulder width. Press
straight upwards as you would a
bar. Pressing with dumbbells
makes it difficult for you to
cheat on the weaker arm.

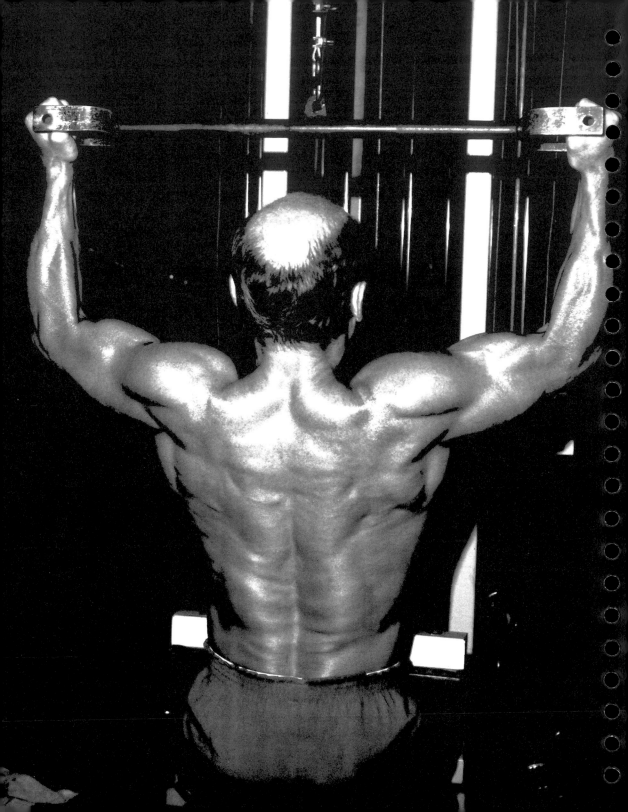

BACK

When thinking of backs, two all-time great bodybuilders come to mind, Arnold Schwarzenegger and Franco Columbu. They have incredible width, thickness, and definition. Arnold thinks that his back muscles are like Conan coming alive and I believe him. Franco's back width is utterly amazing.

The largest part of the back muscles are the latissmus dorsi (lats), and they need to be worked at every angle. The width is worked by doing side-grip pulley pulldowns or side-grip chin-ups. To build the lower lats, you can do narrow-grip chin-ups or pulley pulldowns with a narrow grip. To get at the middle part of the back, do bent-over parallel barbell rows or dumbbell rows. T-bar rows are a favorite of mine and are great for building thickness on the outside part of the lats. An added advantage to doing dumbbell rows and seated pulley rows is that they also build the posterior head of your deltoids, which is usually neglected.

The lower back is usually the most neglected area of the body. It needs to be strong to prevent injuries from heavy lifting. Too many *bodybuilders* have suffered needless lower-back injuries by training with heavy weights overhead without first having built up their lower back muscles (spinal erectors). If the bodybuilder has as healthy back, I prefer starting him out on hyperextensions, first doing them on a flat bench, then later off a Roman chair or bench. I also like doing good morning exercises for the spinal erectors. After having done these basics for six weeks to three months, I then recommend dead lifts. Dead lifts work the legs and the back in conjunction and are a great power exercise. They coordinate all the back muscles in one lift as well as improving your grip, forearms, and traps. I have included stiff-legged deadlifts under the back for simplicity, but they really bomb the hams. In fact, Robby Robinson claims they are the key to his great hams. I do not usually recommend cleans for the bodybuilder because they take so much skill and when not performed correctly can result in injury. However, it is an incredible exercise for strengthening the whole back, and in sports it helps to give you explosive power. Mike Mentzer and Arnold swear by them, but I recommended that if you do them, you should be closely supervised by an expert and start very light to prevent injury.

Especially when I am training mature men, I like them to do lots of back work. Many back problems can be prevented and solved by training. An example of this is the Bob Pure story I mentioned in the introduction. Have you ever noticed a weight lifter who has a great chest but is slope shouldered? The problem could be that he has done too little back work in relation to his chest work. His overdeveloped chest has actually pushed his shoulders and traps to make him appear slope shouldered. Some pulldowns are not enough; he needs rowing and maybe even pulltos.

You will notice that back work will help you swim faster and longer. Back work will also help you swing in tennis and racquetball—it will help you to hit the ball harder and give you a better serve and return. But most of all doing back work will make you feel better and look better.

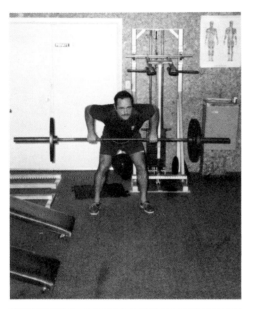

A1: Bent-over Parallel Row
Hold the bar with a wide grip whle you bend over, parallel to the ground. Pull the bar upward until it strikes you in the chest, and then lower the bar slowly. This will develop the latissimus dorsi.

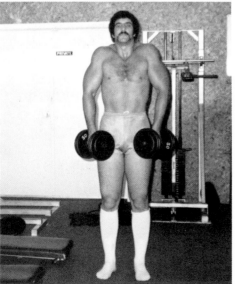

B1: Shrug
Grasp the dumbbells with your palms facing inward. Let your shoulders fall down, and then raise the shoulders without moving your arms.

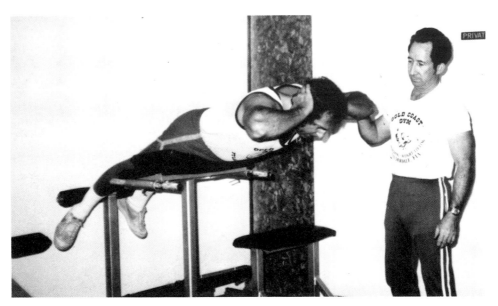

C1: Back Hyperextension
Coach Guerrero instructs his trainee, Bob Pure, how to do this great exercise for your lower back. Go slowly at first and make sure your feet are secure on the Roman chair. This exercise can also be done on a table or the floor (you may need someone to hold your legs).

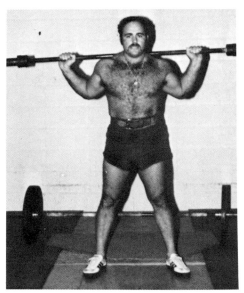 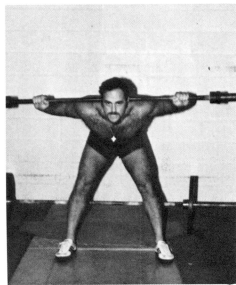

D1-2: Good-Morning Exercise
Start with an empty bar when
you begin and then gradually
build up the amount of weight
you use. Place the bar behind
your back from a standing
position and then bend over
until your back is parallel to the
floor. Be sure that you are using
a light amount of weight to
avoid back strain. Build your
routine up to 2 to 3 sets of 10 to
15 repetitions.

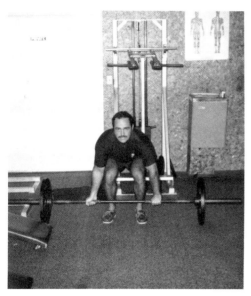 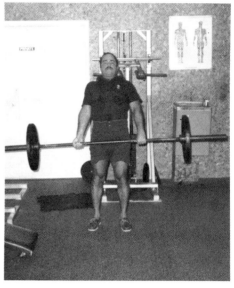

E1-2: Dead Lift

After you have performed the good-morning exercise for a few weeks, move on the dead lift. Address the bar with a grip slightly wider than your leg spread. Hold the bar with one palm foward and one backward. Bend over and lift the bar to your waist, keeping your arms straight. As you get the bar to this position, thrust your shoulders back and your chest out. This should be performed with a light weight for the first few weeks, until the spinal erectors are strengthened. First try 15 repetitions. Then as your development progresses, you can decrease the repetitions and increase the weight.

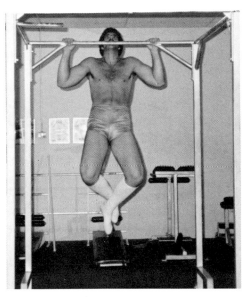 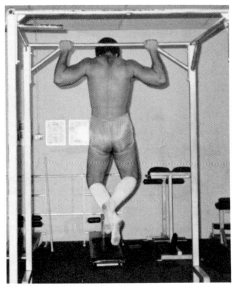

F1: Front Chin-Up
Grasp the bar with a palms-out
hold and smoothly chin yourself
up. Your legs should be curled
or relaxed, but not moving.

G1: Back-Grip Chin-Up
This will develop your lats,
deltoids, and general back area.
Use a wide grip and raise
yourself until the back of your
head touches the bar.

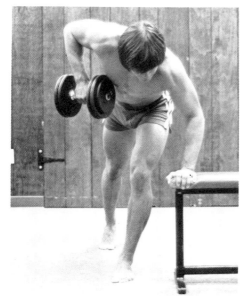

H1: One-Arm Dumbbell Row

Keep both legs stiff and one arm placed on a bench or chair. Extend the dumbbell fully downwards and then lift it back up till it hits your chest. Remember to keep the legs stiff and avoid cheating by bending your knees. This exercise should be repeated 12 times in sets of 3.

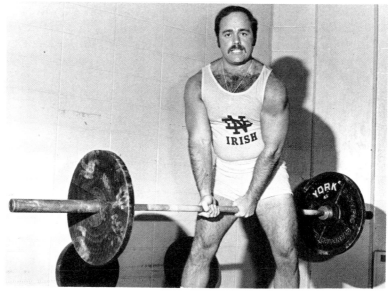

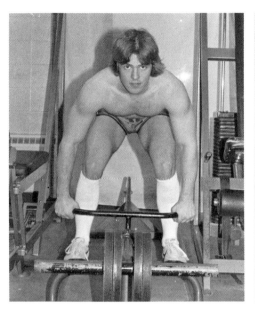
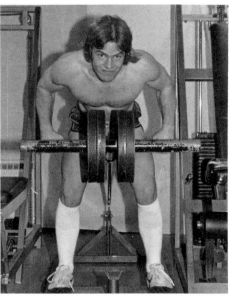

I1: Straddle *(left)*
Straddle the bar as you squat down to grip the bar with one palm up and one down. Then just stand up, being careful to keep your back straight as you bring the bar to your crotch. Then return to the starting position and repeat.

J1-2: T-Bar Row
Upward T-bar rows give the lats more power. Hold your hands on the bar and let the bar drop as you keep your back and knees slightly bent. In a linebacker position, pull the bar up to your chest—being mindful of the full range of motion— letting the bar all the way down slowly and then pulling it to your chest. The form and the motion are more important than the amount of weight. Be careful not to use too heavy a weight at first. Also, avoid using your back—just the pulling motion.

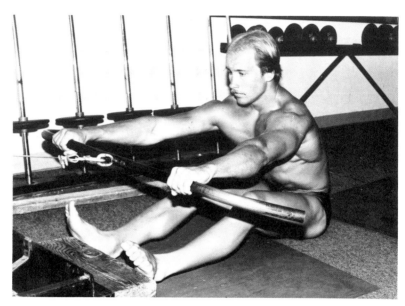

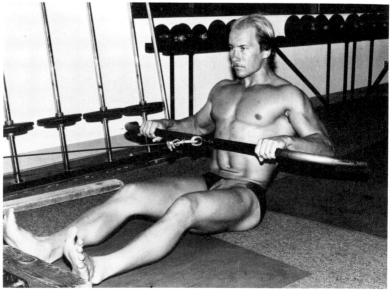

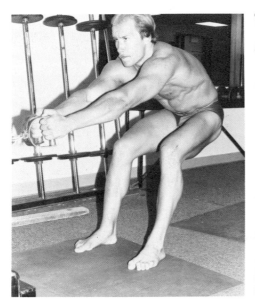

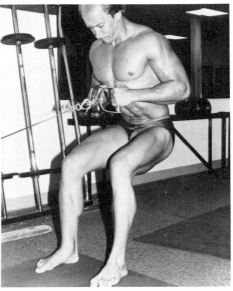

K1-2: Cable Bar Row *(left)*
Seat yourself with your legs and arms outstretched, holding the bar with a wide grip. Pull the bar to your chest and slowly allow it to return to the outstretched position. This exercise will greatly pump your lats and work the posterior head of your deltoids.

L1-2: Cable Row
Stand in a stooped position with a cable in each hand. At a few paces away from the plates, extend your arms fully and pull them to your chest. Return to the starting position. You may also do this seated. As with the cable bar rows, this will work your lats and the posterior head of your deltoids.

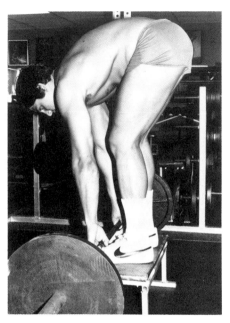

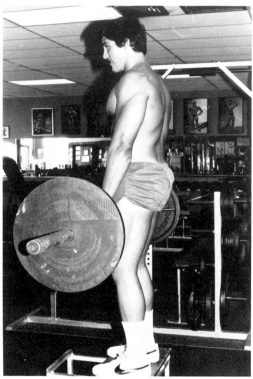

M1-2: Stiff-Legged Dead Lift
Although this is listed in the
back section because all dead
lifts work your spinal erectors,
this exercise greatly pumps the
thigh biceps. Stand on an
elevated platform holding the
bar and with your knees almost
stiff. Bend down till the barbells
go below the platform. Your
back should be at least parallel,
if not lower; then stand straight
up. Make sure you have really
warmed up your back and legs
first. Avoid this exercise if you
have a back problem.

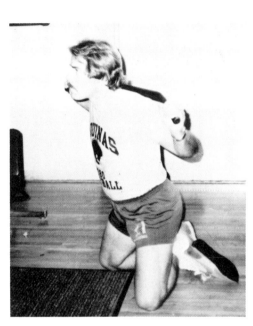

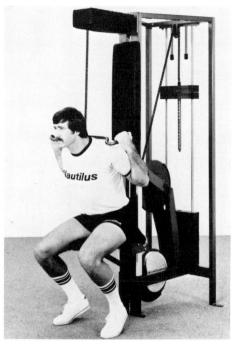

N1: Universal Pulldown
Kneel down with your hands
holding the lat bar at the widest
points. Pull down the bar
behind your neck and allow the
bar to return slowly to the
outstretched position. Repeat.
This is a great exercise for
widening the lats. This exercise
may be done also by pulling the
bar down in front of you.

O1: Nautilus Pulldown
Adjust the seat for maximum
stretch and fasten the seat belt.
Lean forward and grasp the
overhead bar with a parallel
grip. Keeping your elbows back,
pull the bar down behind your
head. Pause. Slowly return to
the starting position and repeat.

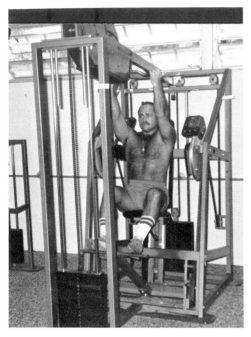

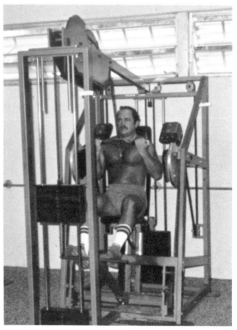

P1-2: Nautilus Compound Back Machine
Grasp the handle with a palms-in grip and pull down toward the chest.

Q1: Upright Row
Grasp the barbell with a narrow grip and raise the bar to a position even with your shoulders. Hold the bar in this position for a second or two while keeping your elbows pointed outwards. Repeat this exercise 12 times in 3 different sets.

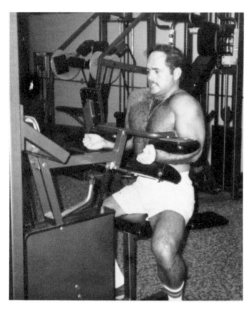

R1: Nautilus Shrug *(left)*
Adjust the machine so that when
you bend your elbows at right
angles while sitting on the seat,
you can place your forearms in
the padded blocks as shown.
Keeping your arms stiff, pull up
by the shoulders.

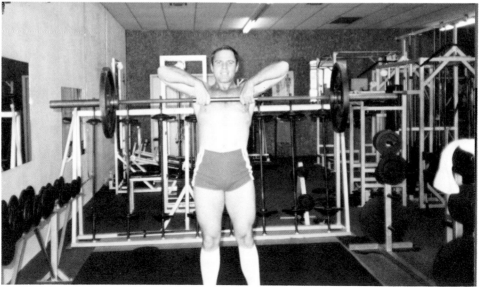

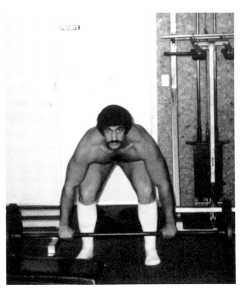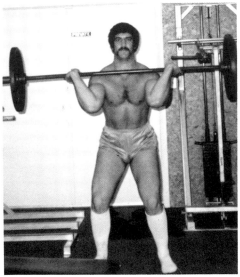

S1-2: Power Clean

With your legs spread to
shoulder width, grasp the bar so
that your palms face the floor.
Your thighs should be almost
parallel to the floor as you
explode into the next position
illustrated. With your elbows
pointing straight in front of you,
spring off the floor onto the
balls of your feet as you lift the
bar to your shoulders.

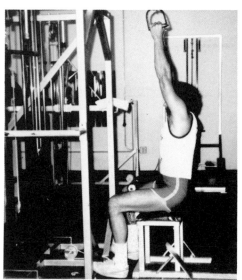 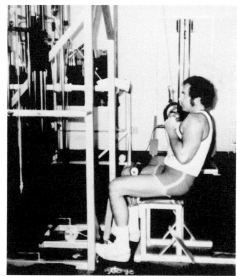

T1-2: Lat Pullto
Sit in the seat and grasp the
rings. While keeping your body
stiff, pull the rings down to your
chest.

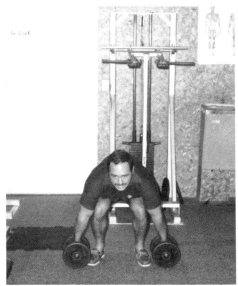 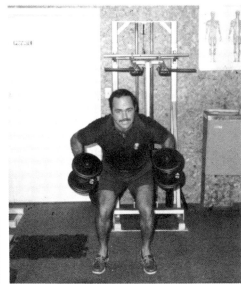

U1-4: Dumbbell Clean and Press
This is the most complete and
important upper-body exercise
possible with weights—an
almost complete body exercise.
Start by crouching in an almost
seated position. Begin to clean
the dumbbells by raising them
over your shoulders. As soon as
the dumbbells reach the top of
your ankles, spring onto the
balls of your feet to complete
the motion. Next, press the
dumbbells either simultaneously
or by alternating arms.

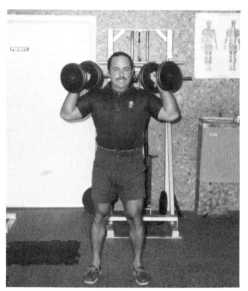
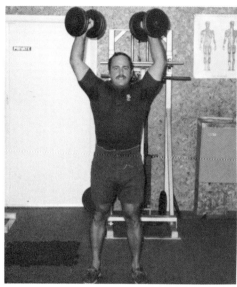

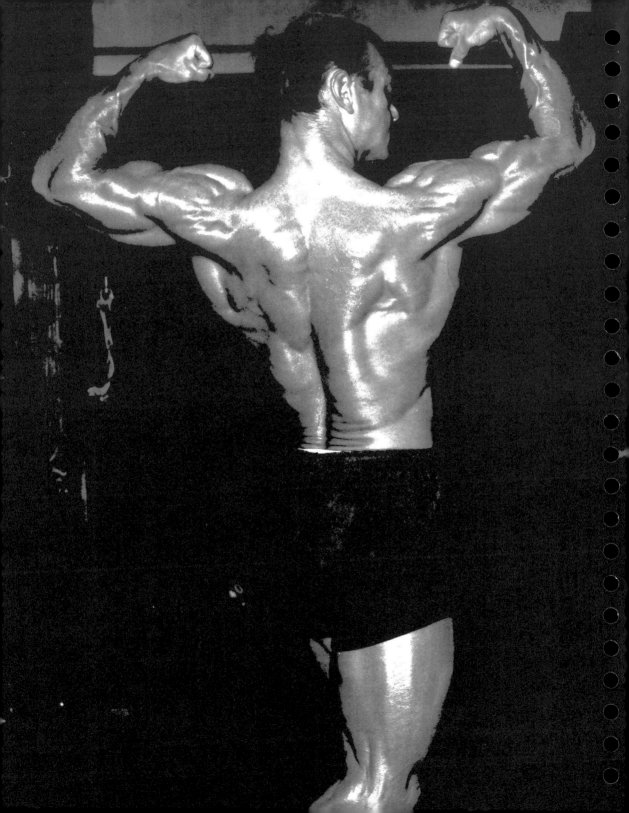

DELTOIDS

"Shoulders make the man" is often heard, and it is very true, since broad shoulders do make a man stand out. Most people are not born with great shoulders but have to work at it. In order to win any novice bodybuilding contest, you must have at least deltoids like melons. Then, later, build them up like banana patches. The deltoid has three heads to it; the anterior (front head), the lateral (side head), and the posterior (rear head). The anterior head is most easily built up because it is worked in any pressing movement. The lateral head is a little harder to work, but responds well to lateral raises as well as a few other exercises. The lateral heads are the ones that make you look broader. The posterior heads are the most difficult to build up and usually the most neglected. You can build them up by doing behind the neck presses, bent-over lateral raises, reverse incline flies and behind the neck chin-ups. When you are in competition form, you should be able to see the definition between the different heads of the deltoids.

Although I have included traps in the back section, you should take note that most trap exercises, especially upright rows also work the deltoids. Any kind of press, whether it is a bench press, incline press, or decline press, also works the deltoids.

For athletes I usually stress the power movements like presses for deltoid development, even though all presses are compound exercises and work many muscle groups. For those of you who are more advanced lifters and interested in working to a super physique rather than just shaping up, I recommend supersetting (doing two sets together that work opposing muscle groups) all the front, lateral, and bent-over dumbbell raises together to blow up your delts. I sometimes also have my advanced trainees superset upright rows with the dumbbell raises or presses with the dumbbell raises. When you first do the dumbbell raises and then immediately superset with the military press, you are again employing the pre-exhaust training technique.

Building up your shoulders will help you hit the ball harder in racquetball and tennis. It will also help you swim faster and give you more endurance. Runners on track teams have been using weights to improve their running for years. Notice the way your arms move when you are running properly and how tired your shoulders get. That should be proof enough that increased deltoid strength will help your running both in speed and in endurance.

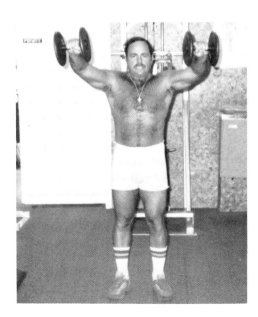

A1: Front Deltoid Raise
These raises are designed to develop the anterior deltoids. Start in a standing position and grip the dumbbells, using a palms-down technique. Raise the dumbbells until they are even with the shoulders and then continue to raise them directly overhead. Be careful not to bend your elbows while performing this exercise so as not to take away from the usefulness of the movement.

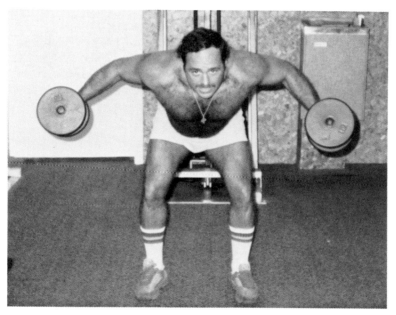

B1: Bent-Over Lateral Raise
The posterior deltoids are the
object of this exercise. Bend over
until your back is parallel to the
floor. Use a palms-down grip to
lift the dumbbells till they are
even with your shoulders.
Conclude the movement by
slowly lowering the dumbbells
back to their starting position.

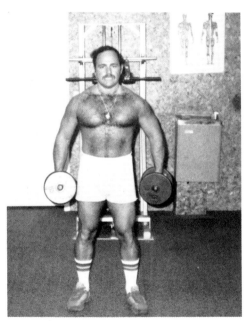 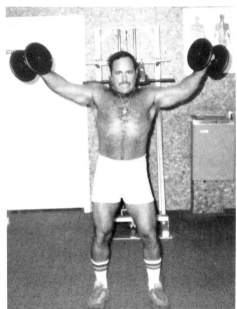

C1-2: Standing Lateral Raise
Stand up with your arms
extended downwards and with
your palms facing each other.
Raise the dumbbells to your side
and above your shoulders. This
exercise does a good job of
pumping the lateral, or side,
head of your deltoids.

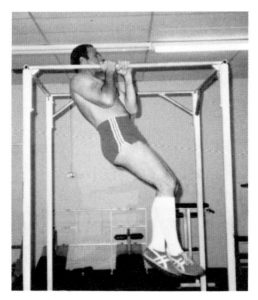

D1: Overhand Chin-Up

This chin-up develops all three heads of the deltoids. Grip the bar with an overhand grip, standing sideways beneath the bar. Pull yourself up until your chin touches the bar and then repeat the chin-up—this time bringing your head up on the opposite side of the bar.

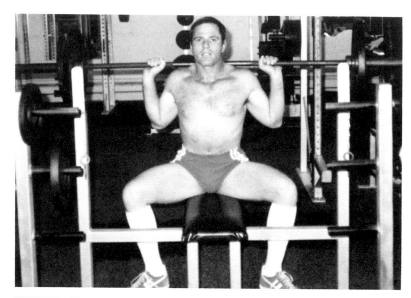

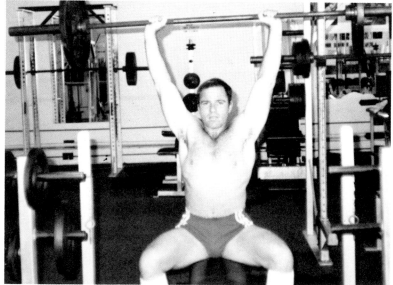

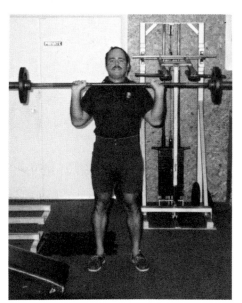

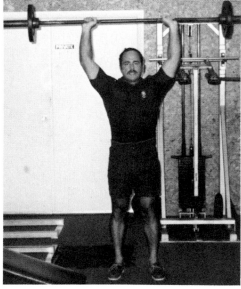

E1-2: Seated, Behind-the-Neck Military Press
The deltoids and triceps are the target of the sitting military press. From the seated position, rest the barbell on the back of your shoulders. Press the barbell upwards, remembering to exhale as you begin your press.

F1-2: Standing Military Press
This variation is similar to the seated press but can be done from a position on the front or back of the shoulders. From a clean position, press the bar straight up from the shoulders.

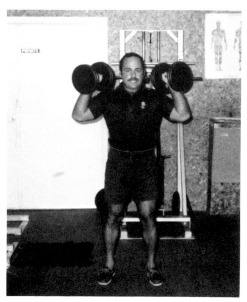 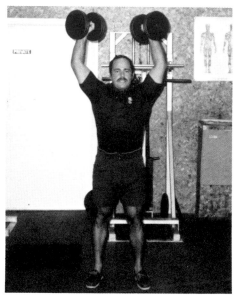

G1-2: Dumbbell Press
From a clean position, press the dumbbells either one at a time or together straight up from the shoulders.

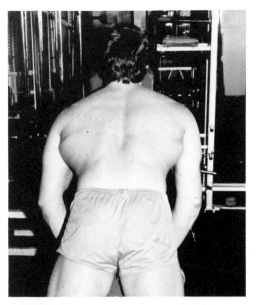

H1-2: Reverse Incline Fly
Lie on an incline bench face
down, holding the dumbbells
with your palms facing each
other. Extend your arms up and
out at shoulder length. This is
an advanced exercise for your
lateral and posterior deltoids.

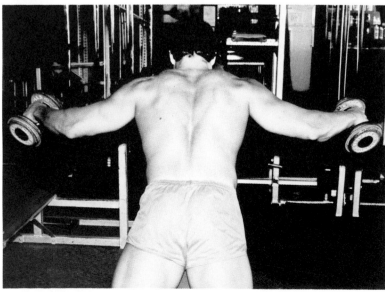

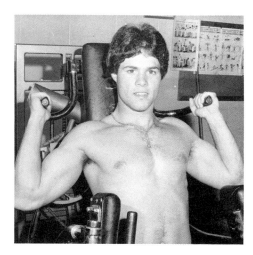

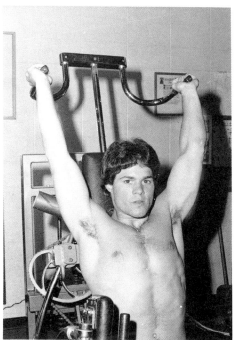

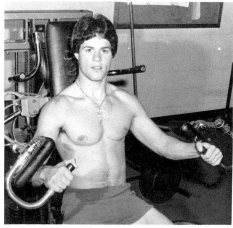

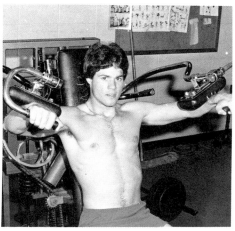

I1-4: Nautilus Double Shoulder Machine *(left)*
Adjust the seat so that your shoulder joints are in line with the axis of the cams. Fasten the seat belt. For the *lateral movement*, pull the handles back till your knuckles touch the pads. Lead with your elbows and raise both your arms till they are parallel with the floor. Pause. Slowly lower your resistance and repeat. For the *press*, grasp the handles above your shoulders and press overhead. Do not arch your back.

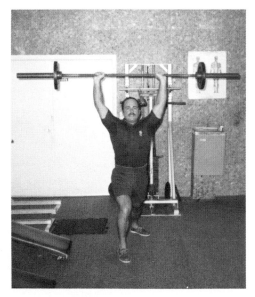

J1: Jerk *(right)*
While in the clean position (balancing the barbell on a vertical line with your shoulders, as shown), thrust the barbell upwards from the shoulder position, scissoring your legs. Then hold the barbell up while bringing the legs together. This is a great shoulder, leg, back, trap, and forearm exercise. It is also an Olympic lift. But be careful; go light. Not all gyms will allow you to do this exercise because it is dangerous.

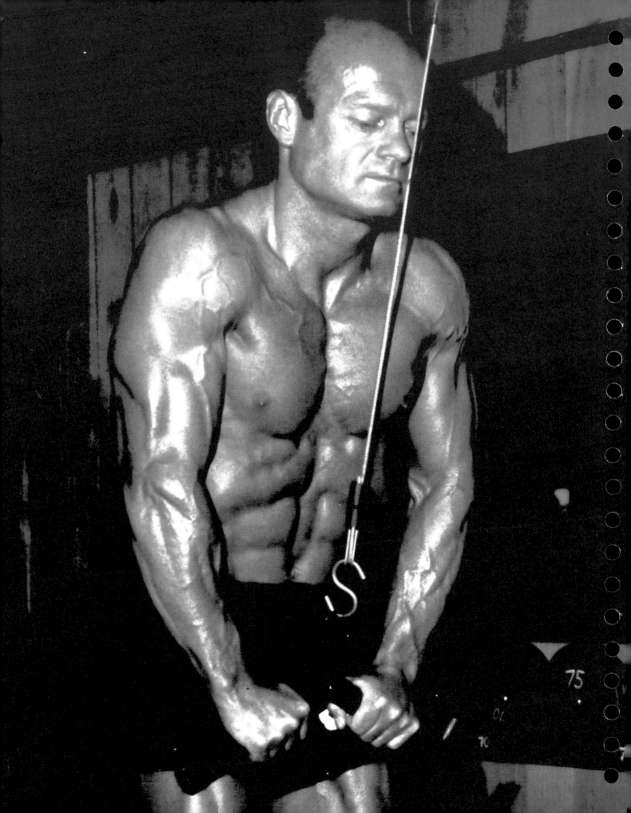

ARMS & WRISTS

Big arms seems to be the most popular item on the training routine of 90 percent of the weight trainers. Most people equate big arms with strength, although that isn't necessarily true. The maximum you can develop your arms "naturally" is based on your bone structure. If you have a six-and-a-half-inch wrist you have a small bone structure, if you have a seven-or seven-and-a-half-inch wrist you have a medium-sized bone structure, and an eight inch or bigger size wrist would indicate you had a large bone structure. Body classifications are also ectomorph, thin type, endomorph or heavy set, and mesomorph or naturally athletic physique. If you have a small bone structure, it will be harder for you to make bodybuilding gains, but you can do it with extra effort. Everyone can't have or might not want to have nineteen-inch arms. If you develop your arms to nine inches more than your wrist size, you will have a decent sized arm. I believe that about the maximum you can naturally (without drugs) develop your upper arms is eleven inches larger than your wrist.

Many people forget that the bicep is only part of the upper arm and that in fact the triceps comprise a larger part of the arm.

The bicep is a two-headed muscle, and when developed to the maximum each head can be clearly and separately defined. Down the center of the biceps runs a thick vein (cephalic). When you train your biceps, you should not only be concerned with size, but peak and thickness through the width of the muscle. Between the biceps and triceps is the brachialis, which can add size to the arms.

The triceps, which are the largest part of the upper arm (60 percent) have three heads: (1) inner (medial) head, (2) outer head, and (3) long head. All these heads should be worked to get that horseshoe look on your triceps and to develop your arm to its potential. The small muscle between the bicep origin and the tricep origin at the deltoid is the coraco brachialis, which is worked indirectly by presses. The forearms consist of a number of cable-like muscles that have the function of pronators, which rotate the head inwards, and supinators, which rotate it outwards.

My bodybuilding programs for intermediate and advanced trainees place bicep exercises along with lats. I, like many others, used to train the biceps and triceps together, but when doing it on a six-day routine, I found I was not getting enough recuperation time. Whenever you work your lats, you also get some bicep work, so I was really overtraining my biceps and triceps. I was also having elbow problems. Combining my biceps with my lats has not only had great results, but since trying this, I have had no elbow problems. These elbow problems were because of all the tricep work. In all presses you get tricep work, so in reality, I was getting some tricep and bicep work six days a week! No wonder the tendons in my elbows were sore. You will also note from my workouts that I prefer dumbbells in my training. Using dumbbells in your curls will give you equal development in the arms, whereas with a bar, one arm will compensate for the other. Doing dumbbell incline curls will give you the stretch that is a key to bicep form and fullness. When you use a barbell, there is a tendency to not only cheat but to get too much deltoid. Preacher curls, which were popularized by the great Larry Scott and often called Scott curls, are great for working the lower biceps. If you have a great peak but no lower bicep developed, you are deficient—get on those preacher curls. However, if you have a problem with sore elbows (tendonitis) avoid that exercise like the plague. If you use 100 pounds on a preacher curl, you have 20,000 pounds of pressure per square inch on your elbows; no wonder it may cause elbow problems. I particularly like concentration curls for peaking my biceps. With many of my other curls, I like doing partial reps through the middle range of motion for peaking.

Before you work your triceps, make sure you warm them up very well. Elbow problems sometimes arise from tricep extensions when you are not properly warmed up. I like dumbbell tricep extensions because they hit all three heads of the tricep. Most of all I like the tricep bench press. I personally prefer pressing movements to leverage movements anyway. The side advantage of tricep (or close grip) benches is that they will shoot up your regular bench, and the pump is tremendous. There are hundreds of tricep exercises, but because of the space limitations I have included only some of my favorites. Remember you get some tricep work in all your presses, so do not overtrain but do hit all heads.

The forearms are worked by doing reverse curls and wrist curls. One of the advantages to doing dumbbell curls is that a secondary muscle group usually being worked is the forearm. Some people do little or nothing for their forearms, feeling that they get enough indirect work from curls, etc. Grip the dumbbells harder, and you get more forearm work.

Wrist curls and reverse curls will help your tennis or raquetball serve and return, but it is even more important for you to develop your arms, forearms, and wrists to prevent elbow problems (tendonitis, which may be called *tennis elbow*, and hyper-extension of the elbow). Runners should also be concerned with building up their arms for endurance and speed. Track simulating the running motion, to strengthen their arms. Swimmers are constantly using their arms in their strokes, and improved arm strength will not only help endurance but also speed. Remember, every little bit helps.

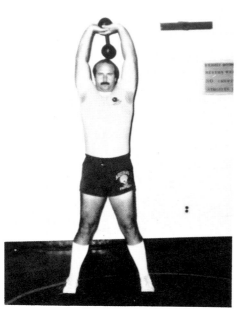 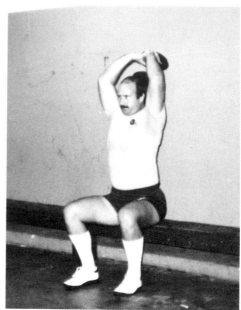

A1-2: Standing or Seated Tricep Extension

Choose whichever position is more comfortable for you. Start by gripping the dumbbell with both hands. Lower it behind your head as low as it will go. Slowly press the dumbbell over your head, making sure that your elbows are pointed inwards as you press upwards.

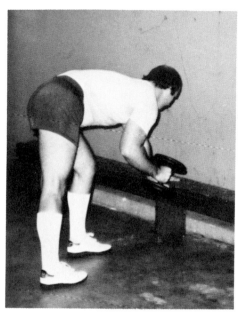 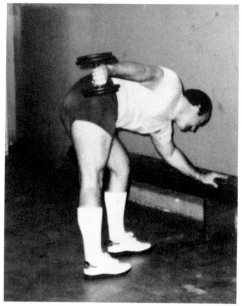

B1-2: Tricep Kick
Bend over at your waist till your
back is almost parallel to the
ground. While holding a
dumbbell in your hands and
keeping your upper arms
parallel to the ground, slowly
straighten your arms back. Then
bring the dumbbell to the
starting position and repeat.

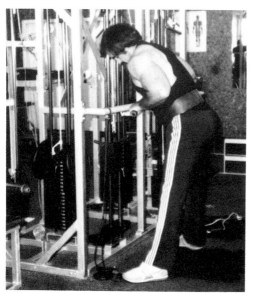 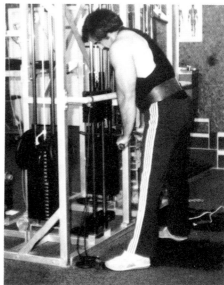

C1-2: Tricep Pushdown
Stand erect, narrow grip on bar,
palms down or up, and elbows
fixed at your sides. Take a deep
breath and force the bar down
till the arm is fully extended.
Exhale. Return.

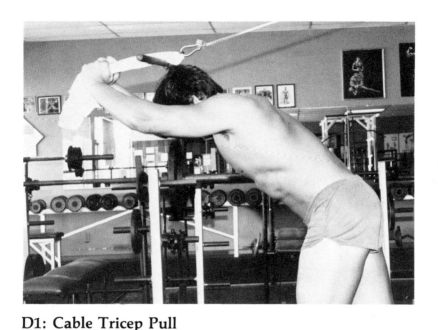

D1: Cable Tricep Pull
Although the model is shown
using a towel here, you can use
a small bent bar if you choose.
Take a few steps forward from
the cable and extend your arms
all the way back. Bring the
towel at least two-thirds of the
way forward, well past your
head. This exercise effectively
bombs your triceps.

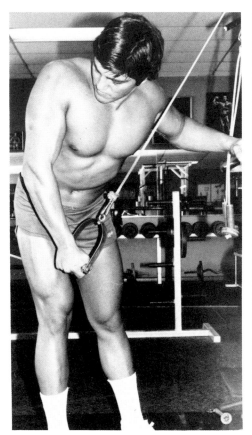 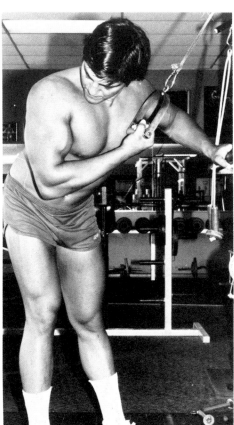

E1-2: Tricep Pulldown
At an angle facing the cable, and while holding the cable with a palms-up grip, pull down till your arms extend fully. Then let the cable return to your shoulder level and continue. This is an excellent exercise for your triceps.

F1-2: Lying Tricep Extension
(right)
In a prone position, grip the easy-curl bar with your hands close together. Hold the bar over your forehead and press it upwards to a position directly over your chest. Make sure you extend your arms completely.

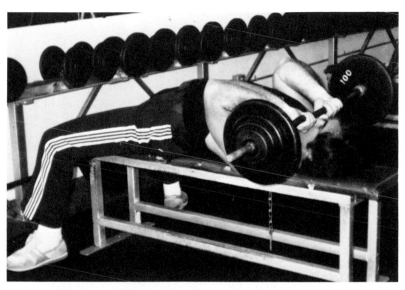

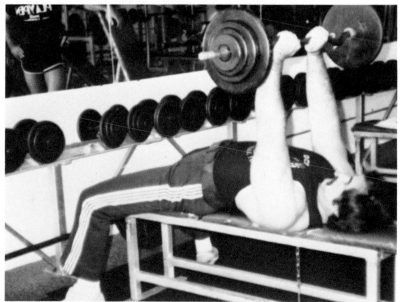

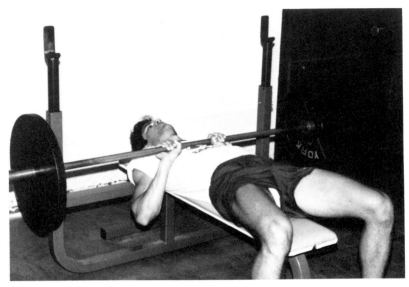

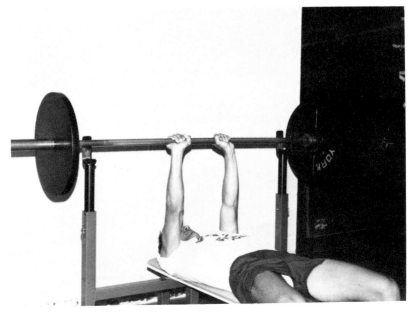

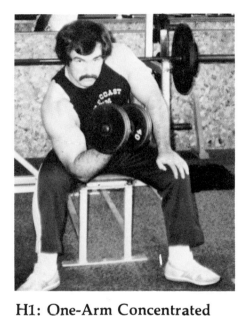

G1-2: Tricep Bench Press *(left)*
This is similar to the regular bench press except for the grip. Use a narrow grip and lower the bar to your lower pectoral area. Keep your back in contact with the bench as you explode the press bar into the air.

H1: One-Arm Concentrated Curl
Start with a palms-up grip. Touch your upper arm to the same-side leg. Proceed to curl the dumbbell until you touch your shoulder.

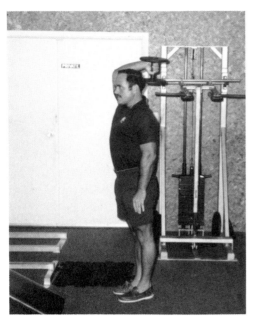 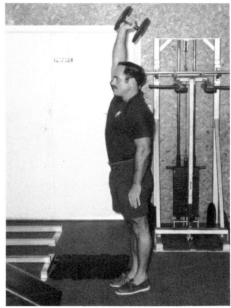

I1-2: One-Arm French Curl

Again you can choose a standing or sitting position. Grasp the dumbbell in a palms-up grip with the dumbbell horizontal to the floor. Lift it over your shoulder, twisting it so that it is now in a vertical position. Drop the dumbbell behind the shoulder, remembering to keep your arm and elbow pointed straight ahead. Complete the exercise by pressing the dumbbell straight over your shoulders.

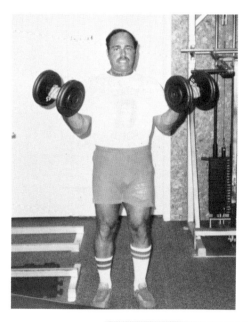

J1: Two-Arm Dumbbell Curl (standing)

These curls can be donewtih both arms simultaneously or in an alternating fashion. Using a palms-up grip from the resting position (arms by your sides), curl the dumbbell upwards and twist it at the hip so that your palms are now aimed at the inside of your shoulder.

K1: Standing Bar Curl

Grip the straight bar in a wide or narrow grip while standing straight. Curl the bar to your shoulders. If you are using a heavy weight, you can cheat by bending your back slightly. But be careful. This exercise puts strain on the lower back.

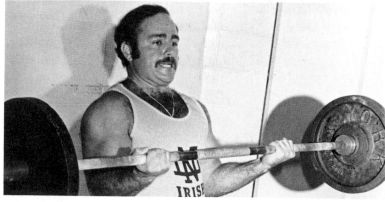

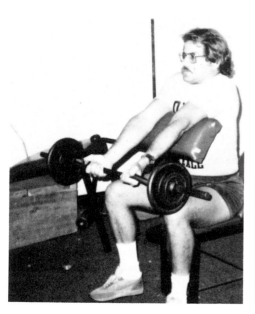 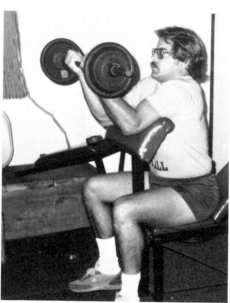

L1-2: Preacher Curl
Rest your elbows on the
preacher bench with the arms
fully extended. Curl up toward
your shoulder. This will fill in
the lower part of your bicep. It
is also called the Scott curl after
Larry Scott, who popularized it.
Avoid it if you have tendonitis.

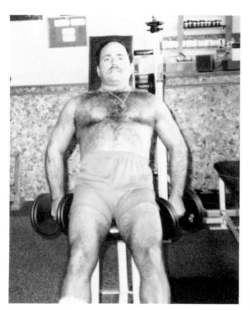

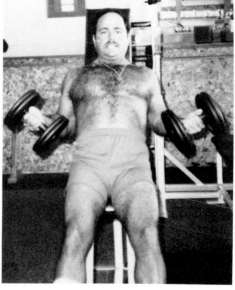

M1-3: Supinating Curl
Lie on an incline bench with your arms extended down, glued to your sides. Curl the dumbbells almost to your shoulders. Make sure the bench is at a 45° angle with your feet elevated. Turn the dumbbells as you bring them toward your shoulder. The stretch you get greatly builds up your biceps.

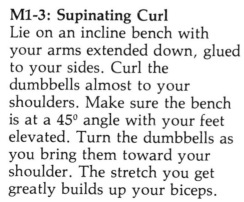

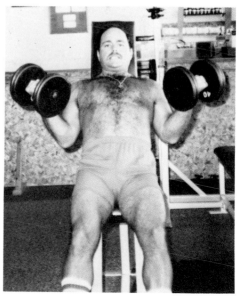

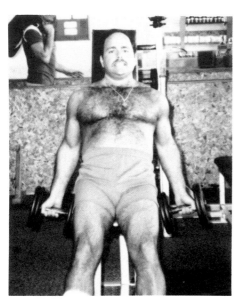

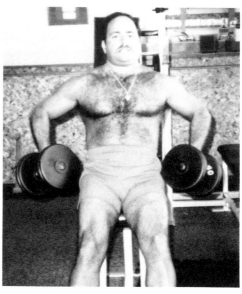

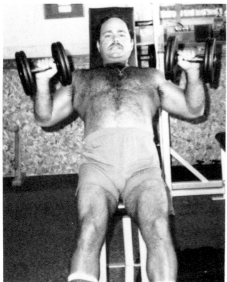

N1-3: Pronating Curl

Lie on an incline bench and hold the dumbbells while at the fully stretched-down position with your palms facing up. As you curl the dumbbells up, turn them at your hip so that when you reach the top of the movement, your palms will be facing down and slightly out.

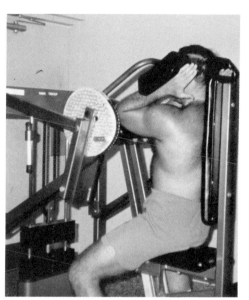 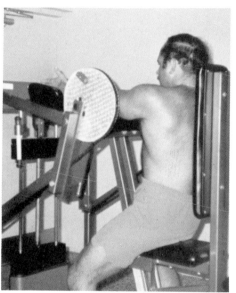

O1-2: Nautilus Double-Arm Extension
Sit in the machine, back securely against the pads. Place your hands behind the pads. Push forward slowly until your arms are fully extended. Allow the machine to spring back into the starting position slowly.

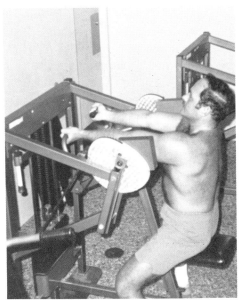 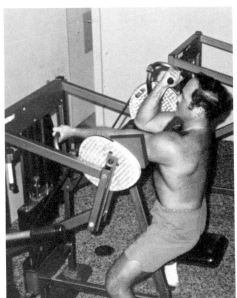

P1-2: Nautilus Double-Arm Curl
Face the machine and grasp the
handles in a palms-up fashion,
arms fully extended and elbows
on the pads. Curl the handles
one arm at a time or both
together.

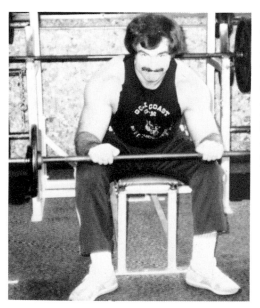

Q1: Wrist Curl (down position)
These curls will strengthen the wrists and forearms. Hold the bar or dumbbell in your hands with a palms-down grip. Relax your wrists so that they drop as far as they will go, then flex and raise your wrists as high as you can.

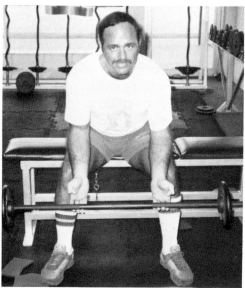

R1: Wrist Curl (up position)
This curl will help the wrist and forearms too, but it adds an extra twist to strengthen the hands and fingers. Rest your forearms on your thighs while holding the bar with your palms facing upward. Let the bar drop to the end of your fingers and then roll your fingers up, grabbing the bar in your palms again. Conclude the exercise by flexing your wrists as high as you can.

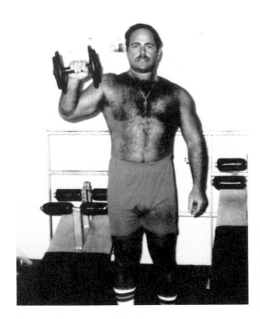

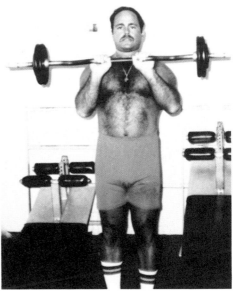

S1-2: Reverse Curl
Take your choice of using either an easy-curl bar or a dumbbell. Holding either with a narrow or wide palms-down grip, curl it to your shoulders. These curls are aimed at developing the forearms.

T1: Dumbbell Incline Curl
(right)
Lie on an incline bench, grasping the dumbbells with a palms-forward position, dumbbells hanging by your side. While keeping the elbow as still as possible, curl the dumbbell to your shoulder.

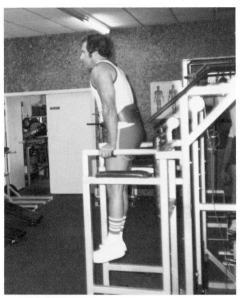

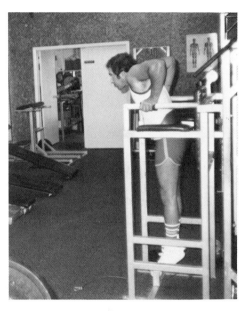

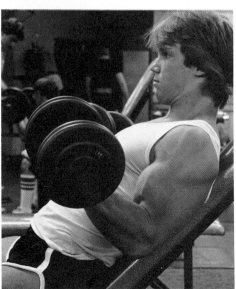

U1-2: Straight Dip *(above)*
Remain straight on the parallel bars and lower yourself till your shoulders and the bars are almost even. Then press straight up till you reach your starting position again.

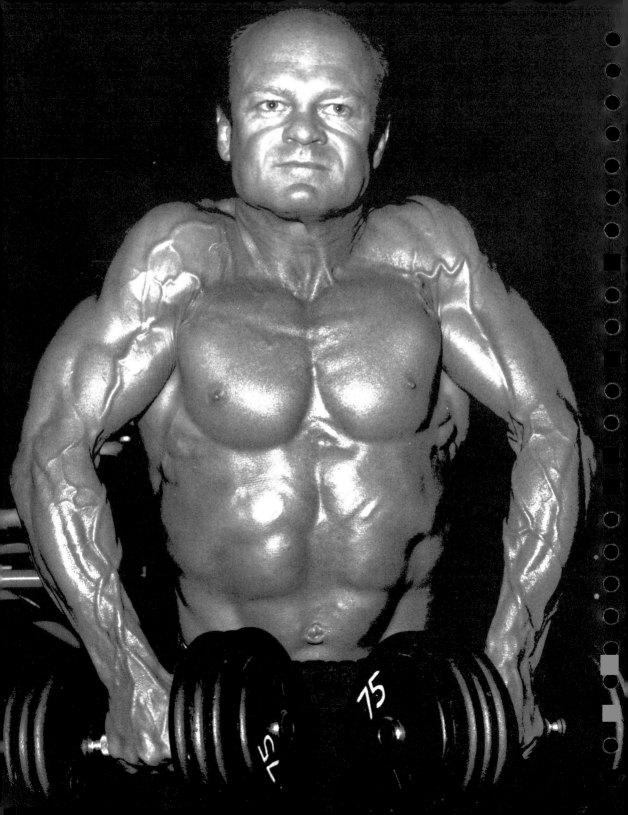

NECK

The neck is probably the easiest part of the body to build up. Whenever you strain, such as in presses, with forced reps, you are indirectly building the neck up. Care must be taken to avoid building too large a neck. Most bodybuilders do not do specific neck exercises because it can take away from their symmetrical look.

For my mature men who aren't still playing those sports that require a big neck, I feel that the indirect stimulus your neck gets from shrugs, upright rows, and the forced reps in the presses are more than sufficient to build your neck up adequately. However, for those of you who feel they have very small necks that don't look good and want quick neck development I recommend either the Nautilus four-way neck machine or the Hydra Gym neck machine. I used both at Notre Dame and at the Denver Broncos and saw some men put on an inch or more in a matter of three weeks. However, tread carefully in this area. Do you really want to have to buy all new shirts right away?

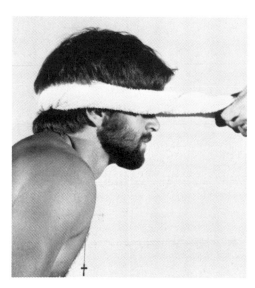

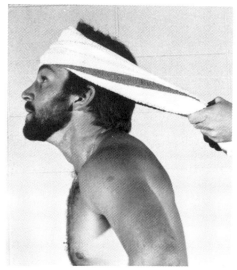

A1-3: Towel Neck Exercise

First start by having your partner place the towel behind the back of your neck and apply pressure toward the front. Try to touch the back of your head to your back while the tension is being applied. Now try the same exercise with the towel on the back of the head and at each side. Attempt to move your head in the opposite direction of the tension, bringing your head forward to your chest or your ear to your shoulder.

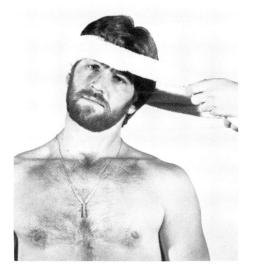

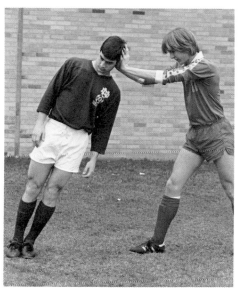 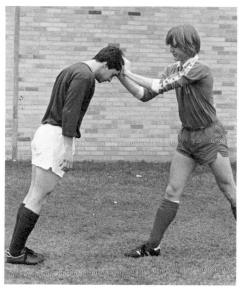

B1-2: Isometric Neck Exercise
This exercise will put constant
pressure on the neck muscles
while the exerciser is leaning
into the arms of his partner. The
neck muscles are doing the work
supporting the person's weight.
Just stand stiff and lean into
your partner, allowing all your
weight to be supported by the
neck muscles. This exercise
should be done in all
directions—front, back, left, and
right.

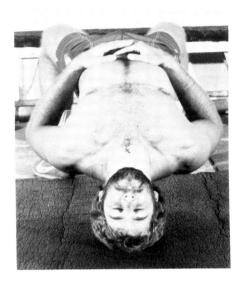

C1: Wrestler's Bridge
Place your feet flat and firm as you bridge yourself up so that your feet and head are the only parts of your body in contact with the floor. When you reach this position, roll back, forth, and sideways to get the most out of the exercise.

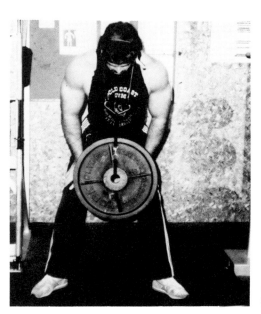 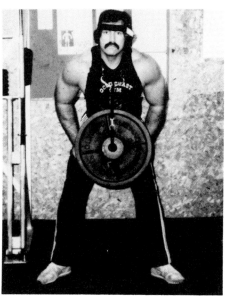

D1-2: Neck Harness
Bend your back as you stand
in a crouched position. Lower
your head and then raise it,
utilizing your neck muscles only.
Be careful not to use too much
weight in this exercise—usually
20 pounds is plenty.

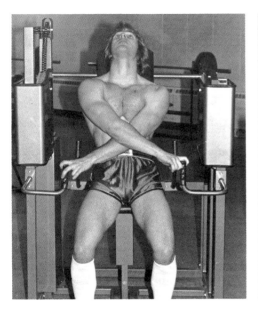 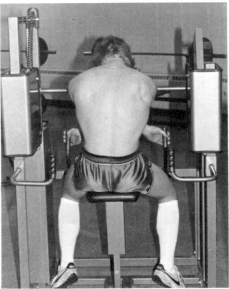

E1-4: Nautilus 4-Way Neck Machine
(posterior extension)
Adjust the seat so your Adam's apple is in line with the axis of the cam. The back of your head should contact the middle of the pads. Stabilize your torso by lightly grasping the handles. Extend your head as far back as possible and pause. Slowly return to the stretched position and repeat.

(anterior flexion)
Face the machine and adjust the seat so your nose is in the center of the pads. Stabilize your torso by lightly gripping the handles. Smoothly move your head toward your chest. Pause. Then slowly return to the stretched position and repeat.

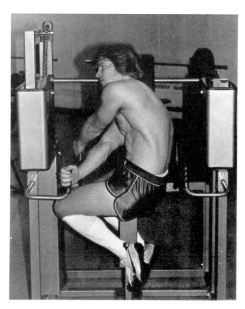 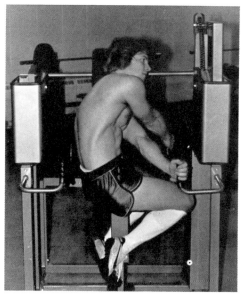

(lateral contraction)
Your ear should be in the center
of the pads. Stabilize your torso
by lightly grasping the handles.
Smoothly move your head
toward your same-side shoulder.
Pause. Keep your shoulders
square·and then slowly return to
the stretched position and
repeat. Reverse the procedure
for the other side of your neck.

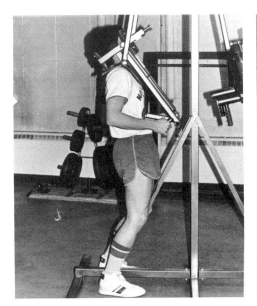
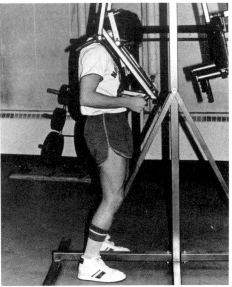
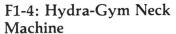

F1-4: Hydra-Gym Neck Machine

For the front-to-back exercise (**F1-2**), place your face about midway of the two front pads and adjust the machine to fit snugly. The chest should be tight against the bottom pad. Push back with the back of the head till you reach the maximum backward flexion. Then push directly forward into the pads until you reach the maximum forward flexion. For the side-to-side exerciser (**F3-4**), place the head about midway between the two sets of pads (you should be able to see just over the bar that holds the cylinders) and adjust the head pads to fit snugly against the sides of the head. The arms should be over the two round bars. Grip the two grippers at the end of the bars. Pull the head from side to side, getting the maximum range while maintaining the body as rigidly as possible.

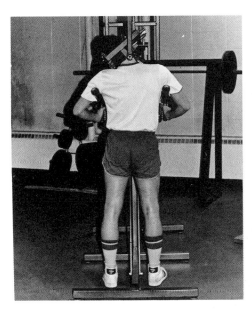
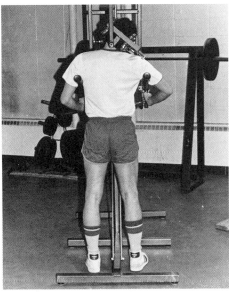

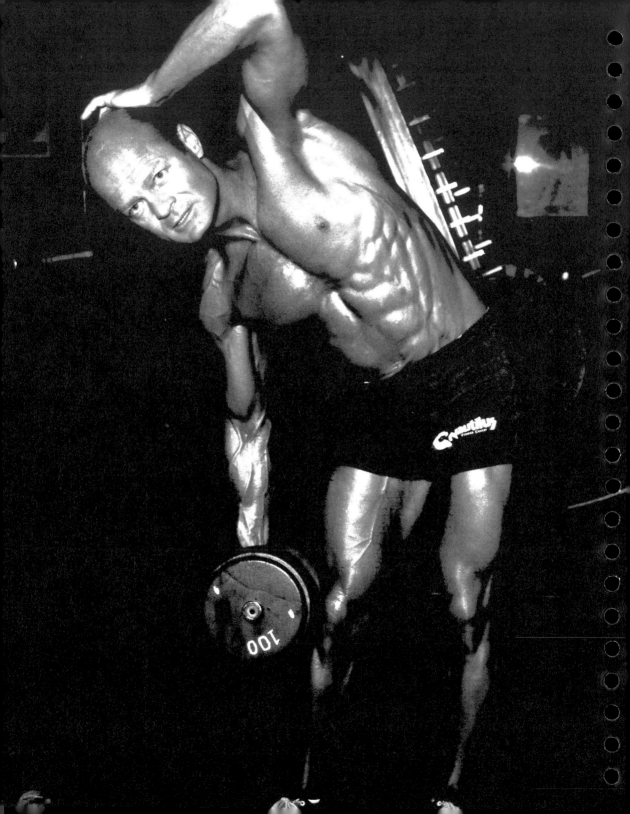

ABDOMINALS

This is the area of the body that most people hate to train but need to the most. Especially for men over thirty-five, this is one of the most important areas of the body to train. That middle aged spread comes way before middle age. You may think wistfully of your earlier days when you had a flat stomach, maybe even with cuts (definition) and you might not have had to do anything to be like that. Well brother, those days are over for the vast majority of us. It is a primary concern to tighten up that stomach. As you get older, your waistline naturally expands, but it doesn't mean that we have to just watch it grow. We can do a lot to keep our abdominals in shape.

You can have a great chest and big arms but if you have a pot belly, nine times out of ten people will say that you are out of shape. Abdominal muscles make the difference in looking like you are fit or over the hill. How can you not be awed by the great abdominal development of Fred Everts? Notice not only his abdominus rectus, but the obliques and serratus inter-coastal tie-ins. Obviously the vast majority of us can't look like that, but we can tighten up an even cut up to an extent. There are many bodybuilders over thirty-five like Frank Zane, a three-time Mr. Olympia, with great abs, and many in their forties or fifties, like Bill Pearl, whose abs can be matched with many twenty year olds. But most of us just want to tighten up, fit into those slacks we bought a couple of years back, and look good.

Next to diet, plenty of work is required to get those abdominal cuts. I have met some bodybuilders who have had great success with lower reps (25) and high-intensity exercises, such as sit-ups on a *very* steep incline or crunches. On the other hand, I have met many a bodybuilder who has success with very high repetitions of basic knee bent sit-ups, elevated leg raises, and Roman chair sit-ups. You have to play your body as an instrument. You are the only one who can *instinctively* tell which works best for you. All of our bodies are different.

Some of the especially good abdominal exercises that I like are angle sit-ups on a Roman chair (it hits the obliques as well as the rectus abdominus), hanging frogs (for the lower abdominals), and the jack knife. You should experiment, trying different exercises for the lower and upper abdominals as well as for the obliques, to see which works best for you.

155

Doing abdominal work is a good way to warm up before you work out and a good way to cool down (along with stretching), after a workout. One stretching exercise, the bar twists, also works your abs. Abdominal work will help your general conditioning, circulo-respiratory condition, and help alleviate constipation. Building up those abdominals is a good way to help to prevent hernias. That should be of special concern to all mature men, not just athletes. You are going to be lifting heavy weights that you may not be used to, so you had better take that extra ounce of precaution and build up those abdominal walls. If you haven't been doing ab work in a while, you had better go slowly. The soreness after just starting to do sit-ups, etc., is quite unlike any other soreness. If you are just starting up, do only ten to fifteen reps the first few workouts, then build up gradually. In fact, ab work can be done every day in your home if you want.

Unfortunately, when you get older, along with the virtues of wisdom and patience usually comes an expanded waistline. Today is not too late to start reversing that trend and obtain a more youthful look.

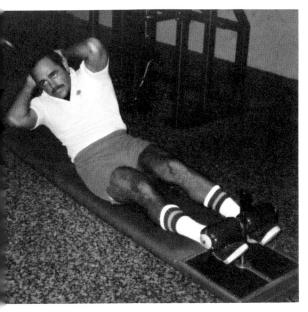

A1: Twisting Sit-Up
This exercise requires a partner to hold down your legs and is aimed at developing the oblique and abdominal muscles. Starting in a position parallel to the floor and with your hands behind your head, raise yourself, twisting as you come up from the level position three-quarters of the way up, to keep stress on your abdominals. The twist strengthens your obliques. This is also a stretching exercise utilized in warming up.

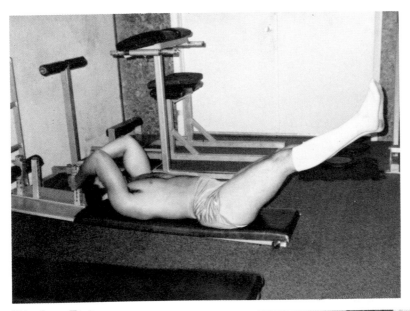

B1: Leg Raise

Raise your legs approximately 2 feet and then bring them down slowly. Do not touch them to the floor. You should do a minimum of 50 raises without stopping.

C1: Incline Sit-Up

Sit on an incline bench or platform and bring your knees up till your legs are bent at a 90° angle. Your feet should be in contact with the bench or floor. Touch your elbows to the knees while keeping your hands together behind your head.

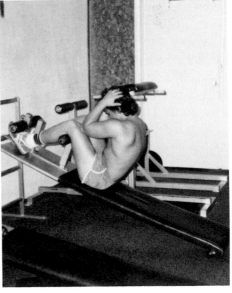

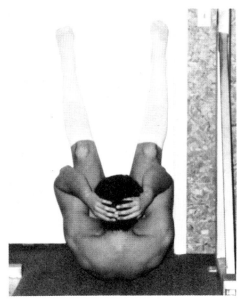 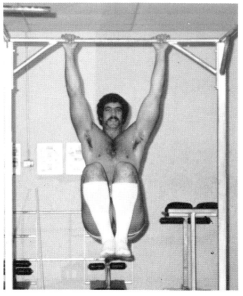

D1: Wall Sit-Up
With your legs completely
touching the wall from the butt
up and your hands behind your
head, try to raise up as far as
you can without moving your
legs away from the wall. This is
a very advanced exercise.

E1: Hanging Frog
Hang straight down from a bar
using a shoulder-width grip.
Attempt to bring your knees to
your chest but don't be
disappointed if you can't do it
completely. It will probably take
a few weeks before you can
bring the knees all the way up
to the chest. Try to stay steady.

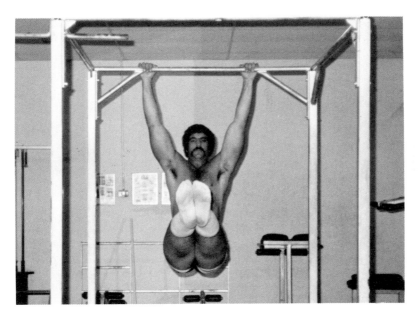

F1: Hanging Leg Raise
Hang from the bar with your
legs together, and then bring
your legs to a parallel position
with the ground. Try to keep
your legs perfectly straight.

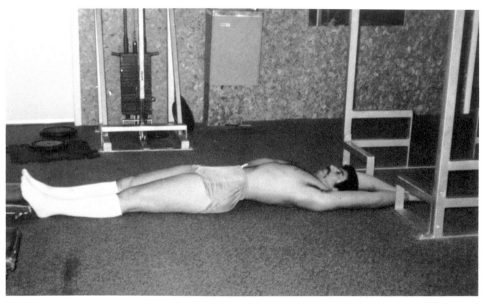

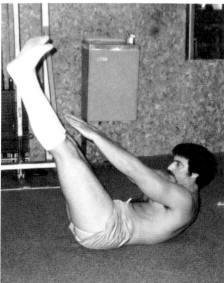

G1-2: Jack Knife *(left)*
This is a combination sit-up and raise. With your arms outstretched and your legs kept stiff, raise your back and legs so that your hands touch your ankles.

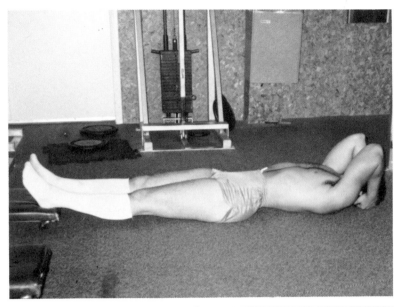

H1-2: Lying Knee Raise

This exercise greatly works your lower abdominals. Lie on your back with your hands behind your neck and bring your knees up toward your chest while bending your legs.

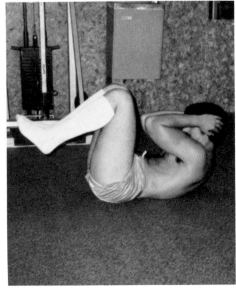

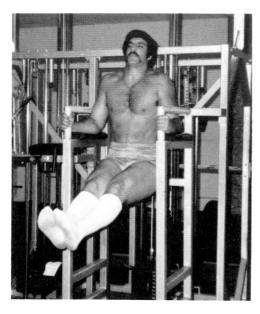

I1: Leg Raise (on knee board)
Rest your elbows on the pads and simply pull your legs up parallel to the floor.

J1-2: Roman Chair Angle Sit-Up
Lie face up on the Roman chair. Then raise up from the bottom position to the top at an angle, twisting as you go up. In addition to working your abdominals, you will also work your obliques.

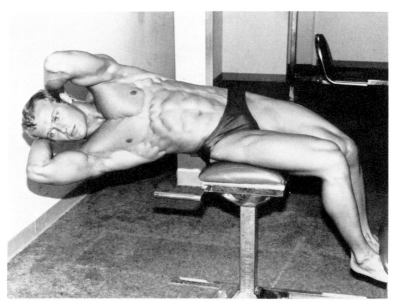

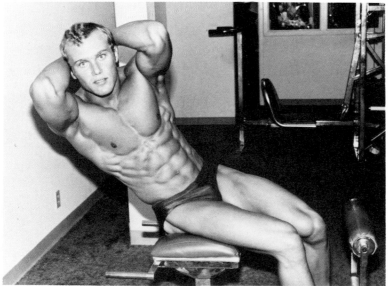

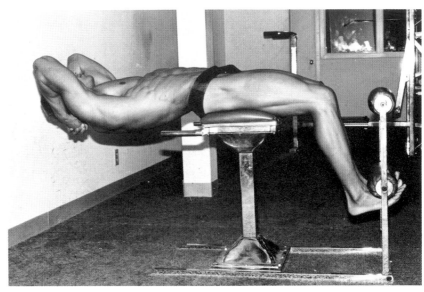

K1-2: Roman Chair Sit-Up

Lie on your back across the
Roman chair, your feet under
the pads as shown. Sit up on the
Roman chair with your hands
behind your neck. Slowly extend
yourself backwards till you are
almost touching the floor. Then
raise yourself up to the seated
position. This exercise will also
work your lower back.

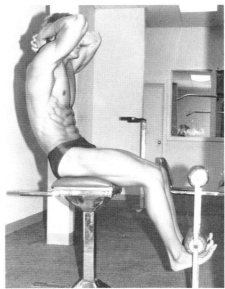

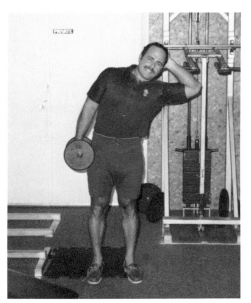

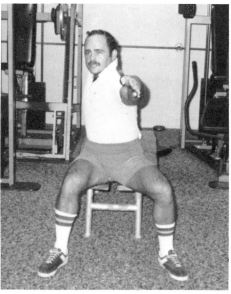

L1: Side Bend
Use a light dumbbell—10
pounds or less—to work the
oblique muscle group. Bend to
the opposite side of the weight a
minimum of 50 times a side.
Don't use too heavy a weight or
you'll bulk the muscle more than
you want to.

M1: Twisting and Flexing
This exercise has many different
purposes. It can be used to
warm up, get the blood flowing,
and loosen up the back and
stomach. Hold the bar behind
your head and twist from side to
side. It will tighten up the
abdominals and obliques. Do
about 150 of these twists to
warm up properly.

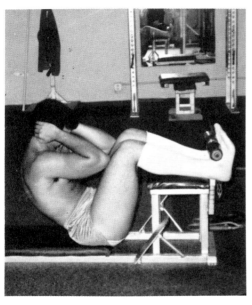 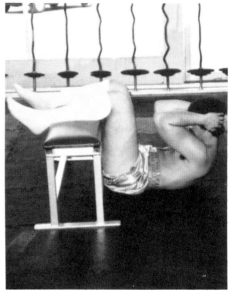

N1-2: Bench Sit-Up

With your legs over a low bench
and your body crunched up as
close as you can get, hold your
hands behind your neck and
raise up as high as you can
toward the bench. You will only
move a little, but this can be the
best abdominal exercise of them
all.

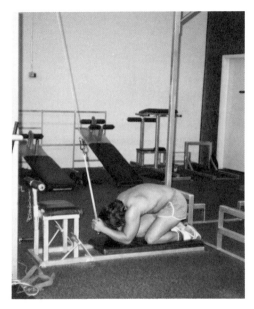

01: Cable Pullto
While kneeling on the floor,
grasp the cable handles, pulling
away at an angle of about 30° to
40°. Hold the cable close to your
head and bend down till your
head almost touches the floor.
Do not move your arms.

WEIGHT-CONDITIONING ROUTINES

Start on these programs only after you have been doing calisthenics for at least a month before starting your weight training. Each session should begin with a warm-up that includes stretching with a bar *(Flexibility P)*, leg stretches *(Flexibility O)*, and sit-ups (see *Abdominals* section). Each session should conclude with a cool-down with stretches, side bends (**Abdominals L**), and a variety of other abdominal exercises.

General Fitness
Beginning Weight-Training Program

Do the following every other day, 3 days weekly. During the first week of training, do just 1 set of each exercise; the second week, do 2 sets; and in the third week, you can do all the recommended sets.

1. 1 set of leg extensions (**Legs A**), 12 reps.
2. 1 set of leg curls (**Legs B**), 12 reps.
3. 3 sets of squats (**Legs G**): use a very light set (50 percent of what you estimate your maximum) for the 1st set, 12 reps.; on the 2d and 3d sets, do 75 percent of maximum, 8 reps. Avoid this exercise if you have knee problems until you consult with a doctor.
4. 3 sets of donkey toe raises (**Legs L**), 10 burning reps. (start counting only after the burning begins).
5. 3 sets of bench presses (**Chest A**): 1st set at 50 percent of maximum, 12 reps.; 2d and 3d sets at 75 percent of maximum, 8 reps.

6. 3 sets of flat flies (**Chest J**), 12 reps.
7. 3 sets of dumbbell incline presses (**Chest E**), 8-12 reps.
8. 3 sets of lat pulldowns (**Back N or O**), 12 reps. or chin-ups (**Back F or G**) if you can do at least 10.
9. 3 sets of seated military presses (**Deltoids E**), preferably with dumbbells, 8-12 reps.
10. 3 sets of curls (any kind in **Arms & Wrists** section), 8 reps.
11. 3 sets of tricep extensions (**Arms & Wrists A or F**), 8-12 reps., or, if you have elbow problems, straight dips (**Arms & Wrists T**).

General Fitness
More advanced (after one year,
if you are up to it)

Do the following twice a week, either Monday and Thursday or Tuesday and Friday. You need two complete days to rest the muscle groups used.

1. 1 set of leg extensions (**Legs A**), 12 reps.
2. 1 set of leg curls (**Legs B**), 12 reps.
3. 5 sets of squats (**Legs G**): use a very light weight for the first set, 12 reps.; on 2d set, do 67 percent of maximum, 10 reps.; on 3d through 5th sets, do 75 percent of maximum, 12 reps.
4. 3 sets of donkey toe raises (**Legs L**), at least 10 burning reps.
5. 3 sets of chin-ups (**Back F or G**) if you can do at least 10, or (**Back N or O**), 12 reps.
6. 3 sets of T-bar rows (**Back J**), 12 reps., or bent-over parallel rows (**Back A**), 12 reps.
7. 3 sets of straight barbell curls (**Arms & Wrists K**), 8-12 reps. (make sure you keep your back straight).
8. 3 sets of dumbbell incline curls (**Arms & Wrists T**), 8-12 reps.

Do the following on Tuesday and Friday or Monday and Thursday (alternately with the above routine).

1. 5 sets of bench presses (**Chest A**): 1st set at 50 percent of maximum, 12 reps.; 2d set at 67 percent of maximum, 10 reps.; 3d through 5th sets at 75 percent of maximum, 8 reps.
2. 3 sets of dumbbell incline presses (**Chest E**), 8 reps.
3. 3 sets of decline flies (**Chest L**), 12 reps.
4. 3 sets of flat flies (**Chest J**), 12 reps.
5. 3 sets of upright rows (**Back Q**), 12 reps.
6. 3 sets of dumbbell presses (**Deltoids G**), 8-12 reps.
7. 3 sets of tricep extensions (**Arms & Wrists A**), 8-12 reps.
8. 3 sets of tricep pushdowns (**Arms & Wrists C**), 12 reps.
9. 2 sets of back hyperextensions (**Back C**), 25 reps. Avoid this exercise if you have back problems.

Distance Running

This program is for distance running, not sprinting. Do the following every other day, 3 days weekly.

1. 1 set of leg extensions (**Legs A**), 12 reps.
2. 1 set of leg curls (**Legs B**), 12 reps.
3. 1st year do 3 sets of squats (**Legs G**); after that do 5 sets: 1st set with very light weight, 20 reps.; 2d set at 60 percent of maximum, 20 reps.; 3d through 5th sets at 67 percent of maximum, 18 reps.
4. 3 sets of donkey toe raises (**Legs L**), 10 burning reps (do just 1 set your first year of training).
5. 3 sets of (**Chest F or G**), 20 reps. (do just 2 sets your first year).
6. 3 sets of bench presses (**Chest A**): 1st set at 50 percent of maximum, 12 reps.; 2d and 3d sets at 60 percent of maximum, 12 reps.

7. 3 sets of lat pulldowns (**Back N or O**), 12 reps.
8. 3 sets of seated dumbbell presses (**Deltoids G**), 12 reps.
9. 3 sets of standing dumbbell curls (see **Arms & Wrists K,** but use dumbbells), 15-18 reps.
10. 1 set of back hyperextensions (**Back C**), 25 reps. Avoid if you have back problems unitl you consult with a physician.
11. 1 set of good-morning exercises (**Back D**), 25 reps.

Swimming

Do every other day, 3 times weekly, but never the day before a meet if you are still racing.

1. 1 set of leg extensions (**Legs A**), 12 reps.
2. 1 set of leg curls (**Legs B**), 12 reps.
3. 3 sets of squats (**Legs G**), 12 reps. Avoid if you have knee problems until you consult with your physician.
4. 1 set of bar lunges (**Legs J**), 25 reps. Be careful if you have knee problems.
5. 1 set of ad-ab machine: Hydra-Gym (**Legs D**), 30 seconds; Nautilus, till failure.
6. 3 sets of toe raises (**Legs K**), 10 burning reps.
7. 3 sets of dumbbell incline presses (**Chest E**), 12 reps.
8. 1 set of pullovers (**Chest F or G**), 20 reps.
9. 1 set of flat flies (**Chest J**), 12 reps.
10. 1 set of decline flies (**Chest L**), 12 reps.
11. 3 sets of lat pulldowns (**Back N or O**), 12 reps.
12. 1 set of curls (any kind in **Arms & Wrists** section), 12 reps.
13. 1 set of reverse curls (**Arms & Wrists S**), 12 reps.
14. Since swimmers need stronger abdominals than most people, after the first year do 100 sit-ups (see **Abdominals A, C-D, & J-K**) and 100 leg raises of one sort or another (**Abdominals B, H, or I**).

Bicycling

Do every other day, 3 days weekly.

1. 1 set of leg extensions (**Legs A**), 12 reps.
2. 1 set of leg curls (**Legs B**), 12 reps.
3. 3 sets of squats (**Legs G**), 12 reps. Avoid if you have knee problems until you consult with your physician.
4. 1 set of leg presses (**Legs E or F**), 12 reps.
5. 1 set of bar lunges (**Legs J**), 25 reps.
6. 3 sets of donkey toe raises (**Legs L**), 10 burning reps.
7. 3 sets of pullovers (**Chest F or G**), 20 reps.
8. 3 sets of bench presses (**Chest A**), 12 reps.
9. 3 sets of chin-ups (**Back F or G**) if you can do at least 10 reps., or 3 sets of lat pulldowns (**Back N or O**), 12 reps.
10. 3 sets of curls (any kind from **Arms & Wrist** section), 12 reps.
11. 2 sets of back hyperextensions (**Back C**), 25 reps. Consult your physician if you have a back problem.

Racquetball

Do this program every other day, 3 times weekly.

1. 1 set of leg extensions (**Legs A**), 12 reps.
2. 1 set of leg curls (**Legs B**), 12 reps.
3. 3 sets of squats (**Legs G**): 1st set at 50 percent of maximum, 12 reps.; 2d and 3d sets at 75 percent of maximum, 10 reps.
4. 2 sets of Hydra-Gym ad-ab machine (**Legs D**), 20 seconds; or 1 set of Nautilus hip-and-back machine (**Legs C**), to failure.
5. 3 sets of flat flies (**Chest J**), 12 reps.

6. 3 sets of dumbbell incline presses (**Chest E**), 12 reps.
7. 3 sets of lat pulldowns (**Back N** or **O**), 12 reps.
8. 3 sets of bent-over lateral raises (**Deltoids B**), 12 reps.
9. 1 set of supinating curls (**Arms & Wrists M**), 12 reps.
10. 1 set of pronating curls (**Arms & Wrists N**), 12 reps.
11. Wrist curls: 1 set down (**Arms & Wrists Q**), and 1 set up (**Arms & Wrists R**).
12. 1 set of back hyperextensions (**Back C**), 25 reps. Consult your physician if you have a back problem.

Tennis

Do this program every other day, 3 days weekly, but never the day before a big match.

1. 1 set of leg extensions (**Legs A**), 12 reps.
2. 1 set of leg curls (**Legs B**), 12 reps.
3. 3 sets of squats (**Legs G**) or leg presses (**Legs E** or **F**), 12 reps. Consult your physician if you have a knee problem.
4. 3 sets of Hydra-Gym ad-ab machine (**Legs D**), 20 seconds; or 2 sets of Nautilus hip-and-back machine (**Legs C**), to failure.
5. 3 sets of donkey toe raises (**Legs L**), 10 burning reps.
6. 3 sets of pullovers (**Chest F** or **G**), 20 reps.
7. 3 sets of dumbbell incline presses (**Chest E**), 12 reps.
8. 3 sets of flat flies (**Chest J**), 12 reps.
9. 3 sets of lat pulldowns (**Back N** or **O**), 12 reps.; or 3 sets of chin-ups (**Back F** or **G**) if you can do at least 10 reps for each set.

10. After 1st year, add 3 sets of cable rows (**Back L**), 12 reps.
11. 1 set of supinating curls (**Arms & Wrists M**), 12 reps.
12. 1 set of pronating curls (**Arms & Wrists N**), 12 reps.
13. Wrist curls: 1 set down (**Arms & Wrists Q**), and 1 set up (**Arms & Wrists R**).
14. 1 set of reverse curls (**Arms & Wrists S**), 12 reps.
15. 1 set of either back hyperextensions (**Back C**) or good-morning exercises (**Back D**), 25 reps. Avoid these exercises if you have a back problem until you consult with your physician.

HOW TO CHOOSE YOUR HEALTH CLUB

There is not a day that goes by that I don't see a new ad for some gym, spa, or fitness center. It must be awfully confusing for the novice to sort through all the ads and all the sales pitches in picking what I'll call his club. One club advertises Nautilus equipment, one Universal, another Paramount or Kaiser Cam, still another stresses free weights. How do you figure out which is better for you? One club has racquetball courts, swimming pool, giant TV, and a restaurant. Another club has an old-fashioned gym and some racquetball courts and a track, and still another just has a weight-lifting gym. Which is right for you?

When I was a senior trial attorney for the Bureau of Consumer Protection in the Federal Trade Commission, I was involved in the national health spa investigation and was shocked by the number and type of abuses in the industry. Some of the tricks were to sell lifetime memberships to people in their seventies, get people drunk at a champagne party and then sign them up, or keep them locked in a little room until they signed up. I could give many more examples of the abuses that were rampant in years gone by. Suffice it to say that the majority of these abusive practices have ended. However, you should still be on the lookout for unethical operators. A special note of caution should be taken of new clubs opening up and having very low and unrealistic membership charges. If it's not a national chain with a good reputation, such as Holiday Health Spa, European, Vic Tanny, or some other reputable company, be careful. A red flag should go up if the new operator is not a locally well-known person with a good reputation. There have been many cases where a new club is opened by a stranger to town, offering ridiculously low charges like $50 a year; then, after signing up a couple of hundred new members, the manager suddenly disappears over the weekend with all the equipment.

I hope that I haven't scared you off by these horror stories, but it's best to be prepared to make an intelligent choice. You are going to spend

175

hundreds of hours and maybe thousands of hours there over the years, so put some real time into choosing, utilizing your investigative skills. First try to figure out what kind of facility you want. Do you want to combine your weight lifting with racquetball or swimming and running? Do you presently belong to a country club or YMCA that already has racquetball courts, tennis courts, swimming pool, and track? If you already belong to such a club, then you don't have to waste your money by joining a gigantic facility that offers everything under one roof. I have found that you can get more out of the different sports by belonging to two or three clubs. By belonging to the YMCA, I have racquetball courts, a swimming pool, track, and even a little weight room; and by belonging to the Gold Coast Gym, I have access to one of the best heavy-duty weight rooms in the country.

Therefore, I would first make a list of the facilities that you want, in order of preference. Check into the cost of joining a weight-lifting gym and either a YMCA or racquetball club for just the racquetball privileges. You might find that combining the cost of a good weight-lifting club at about $150 a year and either a $100 YMCA membership or a partial racquetball club membership for $120 a year, you might be better off because you are getting the best out of each facility. Generally, gigantic facilities that are really clubs and offer racquetball, swimming, and other things besides weight lifting may not be the best weight-lifting facility or have proper instruction. Just because they have a lot of shiny new equipment doesn't mean they are the best (or the best for you). Remember that the type of equipment is not the most important reason for joining a club. You could be fit by running on your local school track and working out with neighbors in a garage that has an Olympic weight set and a couple of benches and a squat rack. Don't be fooled by all the glitter and glamour. None of that will make you fit. Fancy equipment doesn't work by just inserting your body in it. You have to do the work; you have to push and sweat.

After you have decided on what you are looking for, the most important thing is to pick a club that has honest management and qualified instructors. You can call the better business bureau to check to see whether there are any complaints about that club, call the local AAU chapter to see whether they have any recommendations, ask local coaches whether they send their boys to any particular gym, and lastly (and probably the best way), ask your friends about the clubs they belong to. If you are new to the rea, ask your old club operator where you lived whether he has any recommendations. If you didn't belong to a club in your previous home, you might have friends that visited the city you are moving to and worked out at a club there and can tell you about it. Word of mouth always seems to be a good route to go. Then after you have a list of clubs to check into, visit each one at the time you would normally be working out to see how crowded it is and what kind of attention the instructors are giving. Check to see how clean they keep the facility, what condition the equipment is in, what are the members like. If the sales pitch is very strong, beware. If it was such a good club, they wouldn't have to give a hard sales pitch. Is the manager helpful? Does he show a real interest in helping you to get in shape? Do the manager and instructors seem to know what they are talking about? If they make unbelievable claims about what they can do with your body, beware. It is realistic to state that you could lose two inches off your waist, lose ten pounds, add an inch on your arms, and an inch on your chest in the first six weeks. But to tell you that you will lose forty pounds and six inches off your waist, and add three inches on your arms and five inches on your chest in the first month is very unrealistic. The manager or instructor should suggest realistic gains for you to shoot for and keep good records of your progress. Does the managment have any awards or trophies for his club? Does he have a reputation in the field beyond the city or state? Is the management well thought of by the other clubs? It doesn't hurt to ask each club what they think of each other. Try to talk to some of the members to see what they think of the club, the management, and instructors. Ask a member if he has any complaints about the club.

An example of why it is so important to join a club that has quality and experienced management is the story of Bob Pure's remarkable recovery under the skillful and concerned care of Rafael Guerrero, the managing owner of Gold Coast Gyms in Ft. Lauderdale, Florida. In 1975, Bob twisted his back climbing into a boat with scuba equipment on. The following morning he experienced lower-back pain and two days later he had an extreme pain in right lower calf area. The orthopedic physician X-rayed his lower back and diagnosed his problem as sciatica, prescribing traction in the hospital for two weeks. He refused the hospital stay and received ultrasound therapy. During the next year and a half, he lived in constant pain that sometimes was so unbearable he wished his legs were cut off.

Bob reports that he had become almost 85 percent immobile and had to fight every step he walked. He refused pain pills because he wanted to know which of his movements caused the most pain and then he could refrain from making those movements. His right leg had atrophied one inch due to favoring the other leg and he developed a noticeable curve in his spine.

Rafael reports that Bob almost crawled into his Gold Coast Gym. Rafael asked for a complete diagnosis from the attending physician before he would allow Bob to start. After receiving this information, he started Bob lying face down on the carpet while holding his lower back and then having Bob lift each leg backward as high as they could go. Then he would have Bob do sidebends to stretch his spine, followed by bench presses with his feet up on the bench. Rafael stayed with Bob an hour each workout and had him gradually begin hyperextensions, using the Roman chair, which Bob feels was the most beneficial in building his back muscles. Eventually, under Rafael's watchful eye, Bob added good-morning exercises, presses, inclines, curls, and leg work.

When Bob started, he was able to do only 40 pounds on his bench press but after about a year in the gym, he benched 265. He realistically is aiming for a 300-pound bench press. At the age of forty-four, Bob is living proof that you can get in shape after forty and that you don't necessarily have to accept the debilitation that accompanies many illnesses like arthritis and sciatica.

This is not meant as a diatribe against the medical profession, nor is it meant to take the place of good medical care. If you have a debilitating illness, be sure to stay under your doctor's care, but look into at least the benefits you could gain by getting in shape and building up those atrophied muscles. Bob's case is not the only time a crippled man was able to build himself up again and resume a life of normal activities. Cases like Bob's have been happening all over the world.

Even though everyone doesn't have a Gold Coast Gym with Rafael there to train him, in just about every medium-sized to large city in the country, there is at least one good club with a competent and concerned staff. It's just a matter of doing your homework and finding them out. Especially in the larger cities, there will probably be a few very good clubs. For many of you, the cost factor will not be important. You want the best and are prepared to pay for it. However, most people today will have to consider the cost factor. What you can afford will be an important consideration. As I noted earlier, the cost of the YMCA and weight-lifting club could amount to $250 a year, but the cost of the gigantic club with everything under one roof could cost from $350 to $550 a year. On the other hand, if you are just beginning and are lucky enough to be close to a YMCA that has good instruction, a well-equipped and maintained weight room, a swimming pool, a track, and racquetball courts, just joining the YMCA might be sufficient for your needs. After you progress and want to get into the weight-lifting part of your fitness program a little heavier, then it may be the time to join a heavier duty weight-lifting club. But make sure that you have capable instructors to train you.

1. List all the facilities you want in your club.
2. List all the clubs in your immediate area that have the facilities you are looking for.
3. Call the better business bureau to see whether there are any complaints about the club.

4. Call the local chapter of the AAU to see if there are any clubs in the area that are recommended.

5. Call the local college and either ask the strength coach, if there is one, or the football coach for a recommendation. If there is no college, ask some of the top high school staff for advice.

6. Ask your friends, if they belong to a club, what they recommend.

7. If you are new in town, ask your old friends and club staff, if you belonged to one there, whether they know anything about clubs in your new area.

8. Check to see whether there are any national chains in your area. Do they have a good reputation nationally?

9. Do the local club owners have any state or national reputation? Does the local manager have a good reputation locally?

10. Has anyone on the staff written anything that was published? If they have, read their books or articles written by or about them.

11. What background do the managers and instructors have?

12. Do the staffs seem competent and concerned?

13. Are any of these clubs making a hard sales pitch or bloated promises?

14. Do you like the members?

15. Ask some members what they really think about their club staff.

16. Ask the other clubs what they think about each other.

17. Are the facilities clean and the equipment kept up well?

18. Check to see whether the cost of your club membership is worth what it provides for you and is what you can afford.

19. Check to see whether the club has won any awards.

20. Last but not least, do you feel comfortable in that club? You want a club that fits both your needs and you can feel good in, not anxious to run out of as soon as you get there.

INDEX

This book has been designed to allow the user to find specific exercises quickly. The right running head (top of the right-hand page) has the chapter names in boldface type. If an exercise appears on that page or the adjacent left-hand page, the exercise letter designation will appear next to the boldface name. Thus, **Deltoids A-B** at the top would indicate that the first two deltoid exercises (in this case, the front deltoid raise and the bent-over lateral raise) appear on the indicated pages. By quickly thumbing through the book, the reader can easily find the exercise he wishes. The index below, therefore, gives the chapter name and letter instead of the page numbers, as is more common in indexes.

Other great training books!

Shape Up for Soccer

by Rich Hunter (Notre Dame soccer coach) & Pete Broccoletti
100s of photos, approx. 224 pp., 6½" x 8½", index, clothbound $14.95, wirebound $9.95

The **only** total conditioning book for the world's most popular sport (the fastest-growing sport in North America).

Coach Rich Hunter's program was called "the best in the nation" by U.S. National Team Coach Walt Chyzowych. And now it is available to everyone.

The program is geared to soccer players at all levels from age 12 to adult. Beginning with the all-important stretching exercises, the program's principal sections include comprehensive exercise routines in running, speed development, inside and outside ball exercises, weight training, skill development, plus special sections on nutrition for soccer players, goalkeeper exercises, youth conditioning, and appendixes in skill evaluation, indoor and outdoor drills, and sample practice schedules.

The Notre Dame Weight-Training Program for Football

by Pete Broccoletti, with Pat Scanlon
180 photos, 160 pp., 6½" x 8½", index, wirebound $9.95

This book is in a class by itself, and its excellent reception from coaches throughout the country proves it. After an initial discussion of nutrition and flexibility exercises, the first part of the text contains exercises by body part; the second part contains specifically designed in- and off-season weight routines by position played on the field.

The Notre Dame Weight-Training Program for Baseball, Hockey, Wrestling, & Your Body

by Pete Broccoletti with Pat Scanlon
222 photos, 216 pp. 6½" x 8½", index, clothbound $14.95, wirebound $9.95

The most complete, straightforward program ever devised for the baseball, wrestling, or hockey player or body builder. The book starts with comprehensive nutrition and flexibility chapters; then it proceeds to give 122 weight exercises, broken down by body part, and then in- and off-season weight routines by sport and (in the case of baseball) by position played. The body-building routines include programs for beginning, intermediate, and advanced students.

Building Up!
The Young Athlete's Guide to Weight Training

by Pete Broccoletti
110s of photos! Spiral binding so you can work with an open book!
192 pp. 6½" x 8½" clothbound $14.95, wirebound $9.95

This is **the** training manual for 12-to-17-year-olds. Specifically designed for growing bodies. Top advice about nutrition and health. Exercises by body part (including body flexibility). Weight conditioning routines keyed to football, basketball, baseball, soccer, swimming, and bodybuilding. Coach's checklist. Player's checklist. Index of all exercises.

Coupon on next page
Available at your bookseller, or order direct

RIP-OUT COUPON

ICARUS PRESS, P.O. Box 1225, South Bend, IN 46624

Please rush me the following books:

_____copies *35 & Holding: Complete Conditioning for the Adult Male*

_____Clothbound $16.95 _____Wirebound $10.95

_____copies *Shape Up for Soccer* _____Clothbound $14.95 _____Wirebound $9.95

_____copies *The Notre Dame Weight-Training Program for Football*

_____Wirebound $9.95

_____copies *Building Up, The Young Athlete's Guide to Weight Training*

_____Clothbound $14.95 _____Wirebound $9.95

_____copies *The Notre Dame Weight-Training Program for Baseball,
Hockey, Wrestling, & Your Body*

_____Clothbound $14.95 _____Wirebound $9.95

Name _____

Street _____

City/state/zip _____

_____Payment enclosed _____VISA _____Master Charge

_____Acc't no._____ _____Exp._____

Indiana residents please add 4% sales tax.